Things I Didn't Learn
In Medical School

Things I Didn't Learn In Medical School

Tough Lessons from a Lifetime of Practice

Gary L. Fanning, MD

Copyright © 2012 by Gary L. Fanning, MD.

Library of Congress Control Number:		2011963264
ISBN:	Hardcover	978-1-4691-4249-4
	Softcover	978-1-4691-4248-7
	Ebook	978-1-4691-4250-0

All rights reserved. No part of this book may be reproduced or transmitted in any form or by any means, electronic or mechanical, including photocopying, recording, or by any information storage and retrieval system, without permission in writing from the copyright owner.

This book was printed in the United States of America.

To order additional copies of this book, contact:
Xlibris Corporation
1-888-795-4274
www.Xlibris.com
Orders@Xlibris.com

Contents

Chapter 1	Introduction	9
Chapter 2	Reality Check	15
Chapter 3	Who Am I?	37
Chapter 4	Wash Your Hands	52
Chapter 5	Respect Your Fellow Human Beings	61
Chapter 6	Communication	72
Chapter 7	Medical Economics	87
Chapter 8	Know the Rules and Obey Them	103
Chapter 9	Medical-Legal Issues	115
Chapter 10	Ignore Your Gonads	133
Chapter 11	There's More to Life than Medicine	150
Chapter 12	Take Care of Yourself	154
Chapter 13	Final Thoughts	165
Chapter 14	Acknowledgments	173

To my grandchildren

Evelyn
Alex
John

And my children

Michael
Mary Ellen
Sarah

And my sons-in-law

Ted
Steve

But most of all, to my dear wife

Arline

> *Before beginning, prepare carefully.*
> —Marcus Tullius Cicero

> *To acquire knowledge, one must study; but to acquire wisdom, one must observe.*
> —Marilyn Vos Savant

Chapter 1

Introduction

I have always wanted to be a physician and cannot explain why. My mother said that when I was quite young, I had a boil on my thumb that was exquisitely painful. So she took me to the doctor, who lanced it. Evidently, I had a relieved and grateful look on my face after he did the deed, and Mom counted that moment as the beginning of my desire to be a physician. Neither she nor my father pushed me in that direction, so any movement toward becoming a doctor must have come from within—until I entered fifth grade.

At the Springdale Elementary School in Tulsa, Oklahoma, my fifth-grade teacher, Mr. Garrett, had wanted to be a physician when he was a boy. As a young man, he fell from a tree and seriously injured his hip, which left him with a pronounced limp. This resulted in his being advised not to become a doctor, because the rigors of medical education and practice were thought to be too onerous for someone with his disability. This was unfortunate because he was vigorous despite his physical limitations and, judging by his intelligence and kindness, might have been an excellent physician.

Fifth grade is traditionally the year when children are first exposed to matters of human health in any depth in the school curriculum. When Mr. Garrett learned of my interest in medicine, he took care to see that I had extra reading material and encouraged me at every turn. An affable man and a superb teacher, he transformed a glowing coal within me into a roaring blaze. By the time I finished fifth grade, my desire to become a doctor had turned into a passion.

Having gone through high school and college taking all the appropriate courses and attaining acceptable grades, I was ready to apply to medical school. Nothing discouraged me from my goal, and I was eager to begin my career. My first interview was at Albany Medical College in Albany, New York, and the interviewer was a pathologist named Dr. Alexander. He was a tall gray-haired elderly gentleman wearing a spotless starched white lab coat over his shirt and tie. He had a serious, almost-grim demeanor.

I listened carefully to his first question: "Fanning, why do you want to be a doctor?" As the sweat began to bead and my pulse began to race, I told him the truth: my wanting to be a doctor was something that preceded my memory, and I could not recall ever wanting to do anything else.

His reply: "In other words, Fanning, your desire to become a physician is a childish whim to which you have never given a moment of rational thought."

Those were his exact words, undoubtedly remembered after all these years because they are branded somewhere on one of my cerebral hemispheres and because there was at least a modicum of truth in what he said. I went on to explain how I had prepared myself for medical school by studying hard and majoring in biology, a science that greatly interested me. I fumbled on for a while and was most relieved when this trial ended. The second interviewer (whose name I do not remember) was benign by comparison, and he pleasantly tried to convince me to attend that school instead of any other. I think back on it as a "bad cop, good cop" experience. I did get accepted there, but I chose to attend the State University of New York Upstate Medical Center in Syracuse.

Why am I telling you all this? Sitting here at seventy-one years of age, I have practiced medicine for more than forty-five years and still cannot tell you with any certainty why I wanted to become a doctor. From my perspective, it feels like my profession chose me instead of the other way around, so I consider it a calling instead of a choice. Mind you, this does not make me any better or any worse than other members of my profession; it is simply that, like all of us, my life's experiences will color everything I believe and write. I have a passion for medicine bordering on religion, another facet of my being that influences my outlook. You would be wise to remember that as you read. Because of my pride in my calling, I have expectations for the members of the medical profession that others may not share. I find it difficult to accept behavior in a physician or any other health care professional that is anything less than honest, moral, legal, and selfless. To many, that makes me a stuffed shirt or worse. I can live with that.

This book is written primarily for those in the health care professions, especially those about to enter their training; however, people already in training or recently graduated might find it interesting as well. Laypersons not associated with medicine but with a general interest in the field might enjoy some of the stories, philosophy, morality, politics, and controversies contained in the work, because much of what I have to say is equally applicable to people working in other fields. The tone of the book will be conversational, because I want you to feel that I am speaking directly to you. Try to imagine our sitting together, having a cup of coffee and discussing the issues I raise. I love to talk, argue, and reminisce. So just consider this reading as a one-sided conversation. Grab a nice cappuccino to enjoy as I give you words of advice, a memoir, a guide to practice and life, and a compilation of strongly held beliefs and homespun philosophies. There will also be criticism of situations and behaviors I find unacceptable. You will read a number of stories from my life, which I hope you will find interesting. They all happened as I describe them to the best of my recollection.

I am not afraid to say what is on my mind, and if anyone with a critical eye ever reads this book, my opinions will suffer the majority of the artillery shots. So be it. I am not ashamed of them, most of which have been formed after careful thought, study, observation, experience (including both failures and triumphs), debates, and consultation. I am willing to change my attitudes based on new facts or changing circumstances; however, my principles are immutable, forged over a lifetime and battle tested. I am well aware that if a man can find agreement with his opinions 50.001 percent of the time, he is lucky indeed, and I have many friends who disagree with some of mine. I love to spout off, and I will sound preachy some of the time (another sure target of criticism), but not in a truly religious sense. Any morality discussed will be mostly in social or secular terms, even though secular mores and religious mores are often inseparable. I will even quote a religious source or two; nevertheless, I am quite content with your finding your own religion and will not proselytize.

You will learn that I am a practicing Episcopalian and am quite serious about my faith, another factor that greatly influences how I view life and how I react to others.

I hope you read the preceding paragraph carefully. I do not wish you to become angry with me if you disagree with my opinions. You have every right to opinions of your own, and if yours don't always jibe with mine, that's OK. It will make me supremely happy if in reading what I write, you are motivated to examine your own views concerning a variety of issues. I have never met anyone who has all the right answers about everything, not even that guy I see in the mirror every morning when I shave. So feel free to disagree, but let's remain friends.

Why have I written this book? I wanted to share some of my life's experiences and strong feelings with friends and family, and it occurred to me that these might be of interest to people entering medical fields. I also thought about many of my encounters in recent years with young physicians just out of training, some of whom are terrific—skilled, dedicated, and ethical. Others, quite honestly, have a view of life that is so far from mine as to be upsetting, especially in the areas of morality, professionalism, work ethic, greed, and compassion (primarily a lack thereof). I wondered, therefore, if medical school training is perhaps lax in exploring these subjects and if it might be worthwhile to add my voice to those attempting to insert some humanitarian issues into the curriculum.

The ultimate goal, of course, is to produce health care providers who are not only scientifically and technically competent, but also humane, sympathetic, and moral, because the true measure of a physician is not only how he or she treats diseases, but also how he or she treats patients. I do not remember hearing a lot of "thou shalt" and "thou shalt not" statements from my professors in medical school. That's OK in many respects, because medical schools and institutions training other health care professionals are not seminaries. Nonetheless, in the practice of our various disciplines within medicine, some behaviors are acceptable and some are not; and that applies to the perspectives of one's colleagues, one's patients, and society in general. The way in which we conduct ourselves reflects on us and on our profession. The old saw about a rotten apple spoiling the barrel is appropriate, and I do not wish the barrel of medicine spoiled by the behaviors of a few rotten apples.

Those difficult individuals that I have encountered in medicine over the years have left an exceedingly bad impression on my memory. A few years ago, a college friend and I sat in a restaurant after having not seen each other in over twenty years. He is a gynecologist. After the cocktails had been delivered, I said to him, "We worked hard to prepare ourselves to become physicians and have practiced a good long time now. What is your biggest disappointment in medicine?"

He replied almost immediately, "My fellow physicians."

He was right. Even though I have loved and respected most of the physicians with whom I have worked, there are those few who have been the sources of considerable consternation. I have had many occasions to observe both acceptable and unacceptable behaviors, and I have been disturbed that too many people do not recognize the latter. Believe me, I am neither a scholarly philosopher nor an ordained clergyman nor a credentialed medical ethicist. I am a practicing physician, husband, father, and grandfather who has lived a long time and observed a tremendous amount of human activity, which qualifies me to recognize unacceptable professional behavior as much as any person I have ever met. Although I am not blameless in exhibiting unacceptable behavior from time to time, I do not believe that I am guilty of the egregious examples I shall cite.

I wish to leave behind some of the things I have observed and lived and some of the simple values that have made my life easier, more pleasant, and hopefully more appreciated by those whom I have encountered, worked beside, treated, and loved. Those principles have come from many directions and numerous individuals over the course of my life and practice. My few serious regrets have arisen largely from the times I ignored or forgot my core values. Those new age types who disagree with my philosophies and reject my principles will have a field day tossing mud in my direction. That doesn't bother me in the least.

It has been said that it is better to judge a man by his enemies than his friends, and I feel much more comfortable with those who basically adhere to the ideologies I hold dear, ones that I view as mainstream morality. I fully recognize that others will view them as old-fashioned, immature, and naïve; however, I am comfortable with the life I have lived and the moral standards that have guided me.

The title of the book is slightly misleading, because I will include many things that I did learn in medical school, but not just in class or from reading texts. For those just beginning health care training and for those already there, I hope you will benefit from the observations of a seasoned veteran. They say that experience is the best teacher; but it is also the cruelest, least forgiving, and most ruthless. The ability to benefit from both the good and bad experiences of both others and ourselves is one of the huge advantages of being human. As a species, however, we tend to forget or ignore that capability; thus, we keep repeating the same old mistakes. For intelligent individuals who read history and make keen observations of the present, this failing of our kind is a source of madness. No one has adequately answered this simple question: "Why can't we learn from the past?" Actually, we can learn from the past if we so choose. One might define an act of stupidity as doing that which we know we should not do, and our knowing what not to do often comes from observing the acts of others. Unfortunately, some people are incapable of learning from their own or others' mistakes and continue to make bad choices throughout life. Always try to benefit from your own experiences and those of others. It will save you a lot of pain in the future.

For laypersons who read this book, I hope you will gain some insights into the practice of medicine and the mind-set of one practitioner. Being a doctor, nurse, or other medical professional is not as easy as it seems from the layperson's perspective. So perhaps reading this will help you understand and respect your own caregivers a bit more. I am distressed over the stories in the media about doctors and other health care professionals who allegedly do bad things. Without question, there are people in medicine who do bad things, often horrible things; nevertheless, I believe that the overwhelming majority of my fellow practitioners work harder for your benefit than for their own. Mistakes are most often the result of good human beings trying to do their best in difficult circumstances and not the result of bad people being malevolent and malicious. After reading this, despite some of the horror stories I will relate, I hope you will agree.

The physician should look upon the patient as a besieged city and try to rescue him with every means that art and science place at his command.

—Alexander of Tralles

Chapter 2

Reality Check

Is This What You Had in Mind?

Unless you have grown up in a medical family or have already worked in the medical field in some capacity, you have no realistic image of what it means to be a doctor or health care professional; therefore, I thought I might begin by giving you a look at what it is like to be a practicing physician. Forget about what you see on TV. No matter how graphic they make it seem on that screen, it can never compare to the real thing. If you harbor any degree of humanity, some of the cases you experience will brutally challenge your ability to act appropriately and effectively under conditions that would compel most human beings to scream and run. It will be your duty to function at full capacity under such circumstances. Medical training is a good introduction to what you will see in practice, but in the short time of your formal medical education, you cannot see everything. In this chapter, you will read the details of several cases that I dealt with during my career, ones that significantly affected me. Think about them carefully, because they are relatively tame compared with the challenges faced by many of my colleagues as I have heard them described at medical meetings and read about in journals. If you are a medical student or soon will be one, perhaps this chapter will help you focus on your studies and give more meaning to what you are learning. If you are studying to become a nurse, paramedic, or other health care provider, it will underscore how important you are in helping physicians do their duty. If you are a layperson, you are about to read some vivid descriptions of actual situations I have faced. Some of it will not be for the faint of heart, to say the least. It all happened as I describe it to the best of my memory.

As an intern in surgery, I began my rotation in the emergency department at Strong Memorial Hospital in Rochester, New York, on a Saturday morning. Emergency medicine was quite different in those days. There were no paramedics and no meaningful communication between an ambulance and the hospital. Surprisingly, many ambulance drivers and attendants did not even have basic first aid training. In many communities, ambulances were owned and operated by funeral homes, a situation morbidly described by some wags of the era as a classic conflict of interest. There were no cellular phones, and two-way radios were largely confined to the police and fire departments. As a result, ambulance crews simply picked up patients, took them to the hospital, and dropped them there, so-called load and go.

On that first morning of my rotation, ambulance attendants, without any prior notification, brought in a four-year-old boy on a stretcher and dumped him onto an examination table. The child was stiff and unmoving, and his skin was beet red. He was quite obviously dead. The ambulance driver told us that the child's mother found him in a clothes dryer that was turned on and running. In those days, when one opened the door of a dryer during the cycle, the machine automatically stopped but resumed functioning when the door was closed again. Thankfully, this is no longer the case; and now when one interrupts the cycle by opening the door, a button well away from the door has to be pushed to resume the operation. This child had opened the dryer door, climbed inside, and shut the door behind him, thereby restarting the heating and spinning cycles. In precious little time, his lungs were burned by the hot air in the dryer, and he succumbed. His skin was beet red from the heat of the dryer and the abrasive effect of the clothing lashing around him as he tumbled lifelessly inside the machine until discovered by his mother. I feel certain that his stiffness resulted from his muscles being essentially cooked. The vision of that child lying there dead on the examination table has stayed with me all these years. He was sandy haired and handsome, and I wanted him to leap off that examination table and start running around the room. Most people would have burst into tears and run. I could do neither. I was horrified by the mechanism of this boy's needless and most unfortunate death, by the fact that there was absolutely nothing I could do about it, and by the knowledge that I had to go and talk with his distraught parents.

It is heartrending to tell someone that a loved one has died, an emotion magnified many times when you deliver that news to parents. You cannot avoid sharing their grief, and then you begin to think of the guilt and remorse they will likely suffer for the rest of their lives. In addition to offering condolences, you must try to help them in any way you can, such as notifying clergy, family members, and their family physician. Nothing will test your compassion as much as dealing with loved ones at the time of death, especially an untimely, accidental one. Your teachers can do little to prepare you adequately for this in medical or nursing school. While you may be exposed to death and dying many times during your training, it would be hard to train you for every tragic situation you might face in your career. I have concluded that dealing with the reality of death is a duty one must learn to bear, but a task one never becomes completely comfortable performing.

Serious illness and injury in children have been difficult for me throughout my career. I love kids and have really enjoyed taking care of them, but some of the conditions that befall them truly tear at my heart. During internship, I was called urgently to the operating room late one night to assist in an emergency procedure. This patient, a girl this time, was also four years old. Her abdomen was swollen and hard, and she seemed barely alive, breathing in sobs and gasps. When she was anesthetized, the surgeon opened her abdomen, which was filled with blood, and quickly discovered that her liver was essentially shattered into tiny pieces. There were no sizable fragments left to salvage, and control of bleeding was impossible. The surgeon was livid, both because he was unable to do anything to save this little girl's life and because of the mechanism of her injury. It seems that she had been crying, and this upset her mother's boyfriend. After he had whipped her, she continued to cry, so he pulled a nearby chest of drawers on top of her to shut her up. It did—permanently.

Many years later, I was called to help on a similar case, a seven-year-old farmer's son, who was standing behind his father's tractor when his dad lowered the three-point hitch, pinning the child underneath. His liver too was smashed beyond recognition, and nothing could be done to stop the bleeding to save his life. I thought at the time how odd it was to have seen two similar cases; one was the result of intentional abuse, and the other the result of unintentional abuse. Some will think it strange that I use the term "abuse" instead of "accident" for the second case; nonetheless, it was a case of abuse, no matter how unintended and how tragic. Children cannot be responsible for their own safety in the same way as adults. It is our responsibility to be ever mindful of the well being of our kids. Children living on farms have suffered horrific accidents from the beginning of time. Farms in general are terribly dangerous places due to complex and powerful machinery, animals, hazardous materials, and dangerous places, such as silos and sewage lagoons; yet farm kids are found all over the place at an early age, exposed to dangers at an alarming rate. City kids too are subject to all kinds of trauma, which remains the principal killer of children in America. It is tragic that their elders and loved ones are responsible for inflicting a significant number of those injuries, both intentionally and unintentionally. Cases of unintentional trauma are often the fault of parents or older siblings, people who love the victims dearly and who will carry an unimaginable burden of sadness, guilt, and regret for the rest of their lives.

As a fourth-year medical student, I was assigned to a community mental health clinic during my rotation on psychiatry. A mother brought in her three-year-old girl to be seen because of worsening behavioral problems. The psychiatrist in charge carefully interviewed the mother, after which we observed the child at play, a standard technique for evaluating kids of that age. The psychiatrist suggested interviewing other members of the family, including the father, but the end of my rotation came up before any of that happened.

My next rotation was pediatrics. We spent the day in the pediatric clinic performing examinations on mostly healthy children for routine checkups. At night, we took turns helping the interns and residents in the emergency room of one of the hospitals. I loved the clinic because working with the children was so much fun. I used to tease the kids that they had better not touch their belly buttons, because doing so would cause their legs to fall off. None of them believed me, of course, and each straightaway proceeded to disprove that flawed theory. I had the same result with my own children and grandchildren. The emergency room duty was also interesting, but a bit more intense than the clinic work. One night, the little girl whom I had met at the mental health clinic came to the emergency room with her father. The primary complaint was bleeding between her legs. The father seemed quite distraught, and the child was crying inconsolably. The father said that he and the little girl had been home alone, and that suddenly he heard her crying in another room. He said he investigated and learned that she had fallen on a telephone. When he saw blood coming from between her legs, he immediately brought her to the emergency room. The story sounded fishy from the outset, and the pediatric resident was very astute. On examination, he determined that the blood was not coming from her leg but from her vagina. He then confronted the father rather firmly, and the father finally confessed that he was, in fact, responsible for the bleeding. It now became rather obvious why this poor child had been suffering behavioral problems. I am seventy-one years old and have yet to figure out how a father could do such a thing to his daughter. As a physician, I know that the father had his own psychopathology and was in deep need of help to overcome it. Even so, my faulty intellect cannot begin to encompass fully how such a thing can happen. I have concluded that I will never be able to understand it. I have often thought that the specialty of anesthesiology is about as far removed from the specialty of psychiatry as one can get in the medical field. Perhaps that is why I am unable to comprehend this sort of thing. The real tragedy is that this was not an exceedingly rare or isolated case. I am sure you will see similar cases in your practice or training.

I saw many dramatic cases during my residency training in anesthesiology, a few of which stand out in particular. I was called to the emergency room to see a young woman who had just been brought in following a severe automobile accident. As I approached the examination table, the surgical resident was snipping the tiny bit of tissue that had been the only connection between her and her right leg. The patient was still conscious, but only just so and was quite confused about her surroundings and the circumstances of her whereabouts. I had never seen skin color like hers in someone who was still alive. She was pale, pasty, and eerily cold to touch. Both her color and her mental state were indicative of shock, not surprising when looking at her injuries. She had obviously lost a lot of blood, and we began to give her O negative transfusions (universal donor) until we could get type-specific blood prepared for her. One nurse stood at her head talking gently, trying to console and comfort her. Other nurses were trying to clean her as much as possible. Two intravenous infusions had already been established, and a mask was placed over her nose and mouth to administer oxygen. When I looked at the patient's abdomen, I was utterly shocked. The skin and underlying fatty tissue of her entire abdomen had been dissected along her right side and across the pubic area, undermined across the front, and completely folded over to the left where it hung down to the table, like an apron that had been forcibly pulled to one side. The fascia covering her abdominal muscles was completely exposed and covered with grass and dirt, a truly horrifying sight. This was, of course, in the days before seat belts and air bags, and she had been thrown out of the vehicle and onto the grassy shoulder of the road. I could not imagine the forces that had created these monstrous injuries. In all my years in medicine, seeing this young woman thus injured stands out as one of the most visually sickening experiences I have had. We took her to the operating room and spent hours cleaning her abdomen and sewing her back together. We were unable to save her leg, although today with the microsurgical techniques available to us, this might have been possible. She did survive and leave the hospital. Having seen her in the emergency room, I would definitely classify this as a miraculous recovery. I have no clue as to the subsequent mental stresses she must have endured, but I am sure it was exceedingly difficult for her, especially as her fiancé had been killed in the accident.

You never know when you are going to be shocked or from where that shock is coming. As a first-year resident, I was on duty on Christmas Eve. There was a cardiac arrest call to the emergency room to which I responded to find a man in a tuxedo lying on the floor with the medical intern doing chest compressions. I immediately started rescue breathing, and we hooked up an electrocardiogram to find him in a fatal rhythm. We shocked him several times, gave him the appropriate medications, and continued CPR. While this was happening, I asked the intern why we were doing this on the hallway floor instead of in one of the ER rooms. He replied that the ER was full and that a DOA (dead on arrival) and his passenger from an auto accident had just taken up the last two rooms. Because our efforts were totally unsuccessful, we declared the man in the tuxedo dead. As I started to leave, the supervising nurse in the ER told me that the passenger from the auto accident had an open fracture of the lower leg and would be going to surgery. When I went to examine her, you can imagine my surprise in finding that she was my mother's sister. The DOA in the other room was my mother's father. They had been involved in a head-on collision at an intersection. My grandfather, who suffered terribly from arthritis of the hips in a time before total joint replacement was available, had not been able to get his foot to the brake pedal fast enough at the intersection. This was the first time that I had ever met this aunt as she lived a long way from Rochester. She was visiting her father for the holidays. Despite my shock, I helped take care of her for the surgery and had the opportunity to get to know her better as she recovered in the hospital. As I have said, being a physician is not always as easy as it might seem.

A surgical resident was called to the emergency department one evening to see an alleged gunshot victim who had just been brought there by an ambulance crew. When the resident arrived in the examination room, he saw the patient lying facedown on the table with no shirt on and with some blood oozing underneath him. The patient was quite awake and seemingly in little distress. His speech was rather slurred. The resident took out his stethoscope and carefully listened to the patient's chest and then asked the nurses and intern to help him turn the patient over on his back. Imagine their surprise when they turned the patient over and saw a gaping hole over the left side of his chest! There in all its glory was this man's heart in full view, beating away in situ as if nothing had happened. The resident also noticed some blood on the patient's face, and one eye did not look right. As the story unfolded, we learned that the patient had come home rather drunk, precipitating a bit of an argument with his wife. Storming out of the kitchen, he reappeared shortly with his shotgun in hand. After removing his shoes and socks, he placed the butt of the gun on the floor, put the barrel to his chest, and said to his wife, "Look what I can do!" He then pulled the trigger with his big toe. In doing so, he deflected the gun enough that it discharged tangentially to his chest rather than directly into it. This resulted in a large portion of his left anterior chest wall being blown away with minimal damage to his heart and lung. Some of the pellets went to his face, blinding one eye. We took him to the operating room that night, where the surgical team controlled the bleeding and fashioned a covering over his chest wall by moving tissue around from his chest and abdomen. He ultimately recovered.

This man was not the first patient I had dealt with who suffered a gunshot wound, nor would he be the last. It is pretty hard to be a physician in the United States of America without being involved with firearm incidents at some time, either in your training or practice. Some are self-inflicted, as in this case. Others come from lovers, friends, rival gang members, criminals in the act of their crimes, law enforcement personnel, or simply being in the wrong place when someone completely unknown pulls the trigger. Some are strictly accidental, others quite intentional. Gunshot wounds are common enough that we physicians begin to categorize them with appendicitis, strep throat, cholecystitis, and heart attacks: just another common entity seen in America's emergency rooms. The term "iatrogenic" refers to conditions caused by the acts of the physician. Perhaps we need to invent another term, such as "suigenic," to refer to diseases caused by purposeful acts of the patient.

I finished my formal training in anesthesiology in July 1970 and went on active duty in the United States Army. It was near the end of the Vietnam War, and I was fortunately stationed at Fort Knox, Kentucky. This was an extremely active base that provided basic training to newly drafted recruits as well as predeployment training for those headed to Vietnam. It was also a major training facility for officers in armored divisions, and there were tanks everywhere you turned. The daytime population of the base was fifty thousand, and many retired military personnel lived nearby to take advantage of the facilities, including the hospital. In the summer, various reserve units came to Fort Knox for two weeks of training. Late one summer afternoon, I was called back to the hospital because of a training accident. A group of summer reservists was being trained in the use of the LAW (light antitank weapon) rocket, a shoulder-fired weapon similar to the bazooka used in World War II. There was a defect in one of the rocket tubes, which caused the projectile to hang up in the tube being held by a soldier and then explode. The technical sergeant leading the training was killed outright when hit with the largest fragment. The soldier holding the rocket lost the lower half of his right arm and was peppered with shrapnel. Another soldier who had been standing nearby was also showered with shrapnel from head to toe. A third soldier had been hit by a single fragment and had a wound near his right shoulder.

In the emergency room, our first duty was to triage these people to decide who needed to go to surgery first. We had two operating rooms readied and two teams assembled. The man who had lost his arm needed to go rather urgently, primarily to control bleeding. The soldier who had been heavily peppered with shrapnel also needed to go, because he had indications that some of it had entered his abdominal cavity. The man with the shoulder wound looked comfortable enough and was telling us to take care of his buddies and worry about him later. While we took the first two patients to the operating room, one of the fine partially trained surgeons assigned to Fort Knox looked after the third. Because the patient's wound was so close to the chest wall, the surgeon ordered a chest X-ray to rule out any damage. The X-ray demonstrated a long piece of metal that looked like it was going through the lung, past the heart, and into the abdomen. The lung was still inflated. After looking behind the patient to be sure he was not just lying on something, the surgeon ordered another X-ray, this one a side view, because he could not believe what he had seen on the first. The second film confirmed what he feared, and he brought both X-rays to the operating room to show to the chief surgeon. The patient who had lost his arm was the first one finished in surgery and was doing well. As soon as that operating room was turned over, the third patient was taken in. Surgery confirmed the X-ray findings. The long metallic piece had indeed traversed the lung, just missing the heart, and continued on through the diaphragm into the abdomen, where it stopped while indenting the patient's aorta, the body's largest artery. The surgeon put his fingers on the aorta below the indentation and could feel a "thrill," a buzzing sensation arising from the turbulent flow in the aorta due to the narrowing caused by the pressure of the fragment. We were never able to imagine how that fragment missed perforating the aorta, especially with all the movement the patient had gone through prior to the operating room. Happily, all three patients made uneventful recoveries. Those were certainly the most dramatic firearm injuries I have seen to date, but there are many other forms of trauma equally impressive.

On another afternoon at Fort Knox, I was again called back to the hospital because a young boy was injured and needed immediate surgery. When I got to the emergency room, I found the team working on a nine-year-old boy who looked gravely ill and whose color was nearly as bad as the young woman from the auto accident I described earlier. The child was not struggling, as one would expect of a lad his age and under these circumstances. You will come to find it a bit alarming when a child is not resisting treatment to some degree, especially after an injury. The surgeons were working in his armpits, and the pediatrician was placing an intravenous line in his groin. We learned that the child had come running to his house with his arms outstretched, broke through the pane of the storm door, and fell headlong through the broken glass, which cut both of his armpits as he did so. The armpit (axilla) is an important anatomical area bearing many nerves and blood vessels. The axillary artery and axillary vein are quite superficial and large, representing the major vessels carrying blood into and out of the upper extremity, respectively. The boy began to bleed profusely at once. His parents lifted him out of the broken door as gently as possible and stuffed a children's blanket under each arm to stop the bleeding; unfortunately, this simply hid the hemorrhage rather than control it. They drove him as quickly as they could to the hospital, where he received immediate attention. After rapidly gaining control of the bleeding and transfusing the child out of shock, we took him to the operating room for proper repair of his potentially lethal injuries. It is comforting to relate that he did well.

There are times in medicine when you are faced with challenges you have never heard of, read about, or seen. It is ironic that these challenges frequently come after a long day's work, when you are bone tired and ready for both sustenance and rest. After a few years of practice in Iowa, one evening, I was about to sit down to dinner with my family when the phone rang. I picked it up with some dread and heard the voice of one of the general surgeons with whom I worked. "Gary, we have to go to the grain elevator in a town northeast of here. There's a young man up there caught in an auger, and I'm going to have to amputate his leg in order to get him out. I'll need you to put him to sleep." Now here was a situation they did not tell me about in either medical school or my residency program in upstate New York, where they grow very little corn! This was going to be one heck of a first house call for an anesthesiologist. I told my wife that I would not be eating until much later and prayed that there was plenty of gas in our family station wagon.

I went to the hospital to gather up equipment and drugs, my mind absolutely on fire with the thoughts of having to administer anesthesia in the field. We had an empty tackle box in our equipment closet, and I filled it with things like endotracheal tubes (for artificial breathing), laryngoscopes (for insertion of the tube if necessary), and drugs, especially one called ketamine, which is a reliable intravenous anesthetic well suited for people in shock. I knew our paramedics were on the scene and would have intravenous equipment as well as important emergency drugs, supplemental oxygen, and a breathing bag for ventilation. I met the surgeon and his nurse at the hospital; they were gathering things to take also. The surgeon told me that the patient was trapped in an auger in the grain elevator right in the middle of town and that I would have no trouble finding it. Two of the nurse anesthetists that I worked with suddenly appeared. One had been listening to the police radio, heard all the traffic about this situation, and called his brother-in-law, the other anesthetist. Neither of them wanted to miss this event. We all took off for the town, some fifteen to twenty minutes away, driving at a dreadfully illegal rate of speed. I had a citizens' band radio in the car, so we were able to communicate with others of the team on the way.

The men had been working hard all day loading corn from trucks into the grain elevator. When it became suppertime, all but one of the men went up to the office for a brown-bag supper. The remaining man, our patient, set off to activate the giant auger that would transfer corn from the part of the elevator where they had been loading it all day into the so-called big house, where it would be stored until transferred to railcars for transport. The auger ran from one part of the facility to the other and was covered with a long wooden box upon which the workers walked. The patient turned on the auger to transfer the corn and then walked across the wooden box to the stairs that led to the office. At this junction, the stairs were on the left, the wall of the "big house" was in front, and an open alleyway to the railroad track was on the right. Just as he got to the stairs, the wooden box shattered under him; and the powerful grinding auger grabbed his right foot and leg and pulled him up against the "big house" wall, his leg now wrapped completely around the giant screw. He screamed in excruciating pain, but to no avail, because the auger was incredibly loud and because all the other workers were in the office with the door shut enjoying their supper. The machine continued to grind for about twenty-five minutes before someone in the office finally wondered why this man had not appeared. When they opened the door and looked down the stairs, they were horrified. They turned off the auger immediately and called for help. Fifteen or twenty minutes later, our paramedics arrived and realized instantly that there was nothing they could do to get him out, so they called home for the surgeon. About thirty or forty minutes later, we finally arrived.

Once at the grain elevator, we had no trouble knowing where to go because there were police and paramedics directing us to the railroad track area and to the opening of the alleyway that led inside to the patient. Gathering my equipment, I started inside, suddenly realizing that I was walking in corn that quickly reached up to my knees. It was not until later that I recognized that this corn had come from the auger as it continued to turn after pulling his leg inside. Because the corn could not continue into the "big house," it curled up over his back; and taking a right turn, it poured out into the alleyway leading outside to the railroad track. The corn continued to pile up in this fashion for nearly half an hour before the device was turned off. As I struggled through the corn in the direction of a dim light, I saw a young man in a strange sitting position who looked seriously ill. Beside him stood one of our paramedics holding a dim electric light in one hand and a bottle of intravenous fluid in the other. I quickly introduced myself, asked the paramedic some questions about the patient's vital signs, and began to assess this situation.

The French word for "environment" is "milieu." The milieu of the anesthesiologist and surgeon from day to day is arguably one of the cleanest and most pristine on earth. We pride ourselves on a clean environment and in maintaining strict sterile technique. Doing so has enabled us to accomplish things that would otherwise be impossible because of infection. When I worked for an electrician as a youngster, we did a lot of dirty jobs, pulling wires in basements, crawl spaces, and attics. We even wired a complex conveyor system in a gravel pit once, hardly a spotless location to say the least. When I walked into that grain elevator, I was reminded of my days as an electrician. I had not been exposed to so much dirt in years. The air was filled with dust, an extremely dangerous situation owing to the fact that grain elevators have been known to explode when a simple spark ignites this dust. The patient was about as filthy as anyone I had ever seen. He had been working hard all day long, and for half an hour, his traumatized body had been bathed in the dirt-covered corn pouring across his back. I suddenly yearned for the beautiful milieu of our operating rooms.

The patient was frozen in an upright position with his uninvolved leg cramped at an awkward and most uncomfortable angle. There was no possibility of lying him down. You will learn that it is dangerous to anesthetize a patient in the sitting position, especially a patient who has lost a significant amount of blood. This man was close to shock, both neurologically because of all the pain he had endured and because of blood loss. The fluid given by the paramedics was definitely lifesaving in my opinion, and I was incredibly happy and proud that they had been able to establish an intravenous infusion. My pride came from the fact that I had been the one who taught them how to start an IV. Paramedics are wonderful people, and they do a marvelous job with precious little thanks and fanfare. I love them.

When faced with an incredible challenge such as this, I have a tendency to say to myself, "You're just Gary Fanning. How in the hell are you going to be able to take care of this?" Thank God that at such moments, training and experience take command, and things begin to happen as though someone outside of me is in charge. It has to happen that way, because the enormity of some situations is more than a human ought to be able to handle. It does not just happen to physicians. People in many fields, especially trained emergency professionals, often react to unthinkable situations by leaning on their education, skills, and experience. Soldiers in combat rely on their training and reflexes when suddenly faced with critical and deadly situations. Many cannot even remember what they have done in these circumstances, but they have acted swiftly and correctly just as if they were skilled musicians following a complex score. I was suddenly thankful that I had brought plenty of ketamine with me. Not only would it allow me to put the patient to sleep while expecting him to maintain his own airway and respirations, but it would also maintain his blood pressure in the sitting position. Most other injectable anesthetic drugs would cause marked dilation of the blood vessels, a sudden drop in blood pressure, and severe inhibition of respirations.

As I was assessing the patient on my side of the wall, the surgeon had crawled into an opening under the stairs into the "big house." Others had shoveled corn out of the way, allowing the surgeon to get to the auger and to the area where he would be able to amputate the grossly mangled leg. The patient and I were separated from the surgeon by the wall of the "big house." His nurse stayed outside of the opening, but she was able to hand him the necessary instruments and be the voice of communication between the surgeon and me. When all was ready, I injected the ketamine. When the patient was adequately anesthetized, I gave the word to proceed. The surgeon worked faster than I had ever seen him work before, God bless him. Soon, we were able to move the patient away from the wall, and several paramedics and I carried him through the corn in the alleyway. The instruments the surgeon used to clamp off the blood vessels dangled from the patient's wound and provided a strange music as they clanged together while we carried the patient to the waiting ambulance.

I got into the ambulance with the patient and the paramedics. While I was quite familiar with the vehicle and its equipment due to my position as medical director of the paramedic unit, I had never actually ridden in one before. My car was driven back to the hospital by one of the nurse anesthetists while I stayed with the patient in the ambulance. All the way back, I supported his airway by gently lifting up on his thick beard and gave him supplemental doses of ketamine to maintain his level of anesthesia. Mercifully, the trip back to the hospital did not seem to take as long as the trip to the grain elevator had.

When we arrived at the hospital, we took the patient straight to the operating room and transferred him to an operating table. One of the nurse anesthetists had arrived ahead of us and set up the anesthesia machine with all the proper equipment. So we quickly paralyzed the patient, secured his airway with an endotracheal tube, and continued his anesthesia with an appropriate gaseous agent, as we would do for any elective procedure. The nurse anesthetist watched over the patient while I changed into my scrub clothes; and during that time, the nurses removed the patient's clothing and gave him a thorough bath, something he sorely needed. For the next several hours, a general surgeon and an orthopedic surgeon worked diligently to debride this young man's terrible wound, to control the bleeding, and to achieve a reasonable closure.

The man did make a relatively uneventful recovery. He got infected, as was expected, but he responded to antibiotics and surgical debridement and ultimately did well. His mother worked at the hospital in the housekeeping department, and I saw her frequently. She told me that he returned to work and was happy to be alive. A couple of years later, she told me that he had a drinking problem, something I thought understandable considering what he had experienced. I regret that I do not know how his life turned out after that, but I have always considered it an honor to have been a member of the team that saved his life.

Augers are dangerous, but I never thought that I would have to repeat my performance of that night. A few years after this incident, I was about to take an afternoon off after having been on call and working the night before when the call came that one of the surgeons had to go to a farm in the area to help rescue a patient caught in an auger. As I was the only member of the anesthesia team who was free at that moment, I "volunteered" to go along. We arrived at the farm a short distance from the hospital and were led to a big bin used to store soybeans. We were escorted into the structure where we found another venue completely unlike anything we were used to in our daily routine. This time, however, there was more room, a lot more light, and no need to wade through piles of corn, as we had experienced at the grain elevator. There was something else, however, that simply appalled me—flies. I had forgotten that *Musca domestica* is one of the most successful and ubiquitous species on earth and that it could be found in large populations on farms. Here inside of this soybean bin, flies were thick and busy, an annoyance I certainly did not have to suffer on an average day. Then I witnessed an entirely different sight, one that has stayed with me all this time. Sitting on the concrete floor was a woman with a boy about eleven years old in her arms. His leg was wrapped in an auger. Both mother and son looked at me and smiled. No hysterics, no drama, no tears, just smiles. Looking at his leg mangled in that menacing machine and then looking at him in the arms of his mother, I reflected on how important relationships and reactions can be to our species. Had this mother reacted to this accident with horror and hysterics, this scene would have been completely different. Her reaction to this terrible situation was to focus on her son, take him in her arms, and give him as much love and support as she could possibly muster. I was not just impressed, I was extremely moved.

The boy had been helping the hired man to clean the soybeans out of the bin, and they were using a portable auger to complete the job. The lad came too close, and it caught his pant leg, subsequently taking in his whole lower leg before the hired man could get the device shut off. I approached the mother and child as gently as possible and introduced myself. After a few trivial pleasantries, I took a quick history, ascertained that he was a healthy lad, and then explained that I would be putting him to sleep so that the surgeon could get him out of the auger. This time, it was my job to start an intravenous infusion, and it took me two attempts to do so. Again, I used my friend ketamine to anesthetize him; and in short order, my skilled surgical colleague had extricated him from the auger, but at the expense of having to amputate his leg below the knee.

Back at the hospital, we pretty much repeated the procedure we had followed with the patient from the grain elevator accident. We switched to a more conventional anesthetic from the ketamine, and the surgeons debrided and closed his wound. Rather than losing his entire leg, however, this child was able to survive with a below-knee amputation. With a good prosthesis, an individual can be quite functional and enjoy a nearly normal life physically following this injury. He made an excellent recovery and was discharged from the hospital in superb condition. He and his family became favorites of the entire hospital family.

Following his discharge, this boy and his folks threw a party at one of the local motels for all those who had taken care of him. They went to the trouble of preparing special gifts for all, gifts that somehow represented each of our parts in his care and recovery. Mine was a handcrafted billy club that he gave me to use in case I ever ran out of that great stuff that puts people to sleep. It is one of my prized possessions to this day.

This was an incredible family. They epitomized the meanings of love and support. There was no self-pity in this child. Wrestling is a very important and special sport in the state of Iowa, and he became a credible wrestler in school despite losing half of his leg. The grit exhibited by him and his mother on the day of his injury is something that continues to impress me.

You have to be prepared for almost anything when you take call in medicine. Cases on call differ from specialty to specialty, but surprises and challenges are universal. One night, I was summoned to the hospital shortly after midnight for a patient who had been in a serious auto accident. When I arrived, I found the patient in the X-ray department being examined. She appeared to be barely alive, and her breathing was quite labored. While the X-rays were being processed, I performed a brief assessment and realized that she was going to require intra-arterial blood pressure monitoring as well as a large-bore central venous access line. She also needed endotracheal intubation so that we could assist her breathing. As I was about to get the equipment to accomplish these things, some of her X-rays became available. One of them was an X-ray of her pelvis that showed that her sacroiliac joints had been fractured and dislocated. These sturdy joints are at the back of the pelvis where the large iliac bones join firmly to the lower part of the spinal column, the sacrum. Her pubic bones were also fractured. The surgeon took one look at the X-rays and said, "Oh god, I hope she doesn't want any more children!" She also had a severe fracture of her humerus, a crushed chest, and probable intra-abdominal injuries.

The mechanism of this injury was both tragic and interesting. The patient and her husband had recently opened a business and were working very hard to make it successful. They worked long hours, often arriving home late at night. On this rainy night, they got home about midnight, and she got out of the car and opened the garage door. Apparently, the husband's foot slipped and hit the accelerator, driving his wife through the open garage door. In panic, his foot remained on the accelerator, and he drove her right through the back of the garage. The car did not stop until it hit the fence at the end of their backyard. I drove past the property the following day, and the car was still there butted up against the fence.

We spent many hours in the operating room exploring this woman's abdomen and repairing her fractured arm. She spent a long time in the intensive care unit because of all her injuries, but she was finally discharged, another miracle in my opinion. Following extensive rehabilitation, she returned to work and became a successful member of the business community. She and her husband were ever kind to the members of the medical staff who cared for her and returned her to good health.

I do not want you to think that trauma cases alone have impressed me during my career. Certainly, I have been involved in many dramatic ones, but other things have also left important impressions on me. My first clinical rotation as a third-year medical student comes to mind. It was a rotation on general surgery. As I had spent the summer between my second and third years as an extern in orthopedic surgery at one of the excellent hospitals associated with our medical school, I thought I knew all I needed to know about surgery as we began our third year. I was wrong. The three patients I remember most during that rotation were women who suffered from cancer of the breast. The first came in with a breast lump that proved cancerous, and she underwent a radical mastectomy. We no longer do the kind of surgery that she suffered. The operation involved removal of the breast, the lymphatic tissue in the axillary region, and the muscles that lie under the breast. It was a massive, brutal, and disfiguring procedure, but it was also the only one surgeons knew how to do that might have some hope of preserving the patient's life, if done early enough in the process of the disease. We are most fortunate to have less-disfiguring operations and better modes of treatment today, so that this radical surgery has essentially become a historical oddity.

My second patient was a woman who had already suffered this surgery but was hospitalized now with documented metastases of her disease. Having metastases meant that her original operation had not been successful, and that the cancer had returned and spread. In those days, there was no tamoxifen or any other drug that could be used to reduce the aggressiveness of the metastatic lesions. Her treatment was total hysterectomy and bilateral oophorectomy (removal of the uterus and ovaries) as well as bilateral adrenalectomy, all performed to remove the body's sources of estrogen, a hormone that stimulates the growth of some breast cancers. These procedures were considered palliative, not curative. They were not going to get rid of the cancer, simply slow its progress at best. Cancer of the breast is a mysterious and insidious disease that can lay dormant for long periods with absolutely no symptoms. I have seen patients who have been diagnosed and treated for it more than twenty years previously who presented with fractures of the hip that were caused by the presence of the breast cancer in the bone.

The third patient I encountered had undergone all the above and was now admitted with an intestinal obstruction. When they opened her abdomen, it was quickly determined that her abdominal cavity was peppered with metastatic cancer of the breast, and that these lesions were responsible for her obstruction. There was nothing the surgeons could do to prolong her life, but they struggled to relieve her obstruction to make her more comfortable. I became quite familiar with this patient and her close-knit family and learned that she and her husband had been victims of the Nazi regime in Germany and spent a long time in a concentration camp. Their life there had been unspeakably horrible. During her hospitalization, this patient died. I was moved to tears when I contemplated that this poor woman, a loving wife and mother, had survived Hitler's concentration camp only to die twenty years later of a horrible disease that we could not cure. I have ever since hated that disease. Thank God that there are so many things we can do now to fight it. The absolute cure remains elusive, however, and you are almost certain to encounter women dying of this disease in your practice.

There are so many scenarios from my past that come to mind as I write. I have encountered obstetrical emergencies including emergency cesarean sections for fetal distress, postpartum uterine prolapse (in which the uterus actually turns inside out and protrudes from the vaginal opening), and major maternal bleeding crises from a variety of causes, all of which are attended by difficult emotions when you know that the lives of mother and child are in your hands. I have dealt with many young children with acute epiglottitis, an infectious disease that causes swelling of the soft tissues surrounding the larynx, the opening to the trachea (the body's major air conductor), and threatens life by closing off that airway. Thank God that a vaccination has become available to fight *Haemophilus influenzae*, the major causative bacterium of this frightening disease.

One of the most dramatic cases of epiglottitis I ever encountered occurred one night during residency. I was making rounds in the evening and heard a cardiac arrest call to the pediatric floor, something everyone dreads. When I arrived, I saw a whole group of people gathered around the bed of a child who was about eleven or twelve years old. He was quite blue and was having a grand mal seizure. It was virtually impossible to ventilate him, and his jaw was tightly shut because of the seizure, making it impossible to open. I asked for an appropriately sized endotracheal tube and placed it through his nose. Providence was looking exceptionally kindly upon the boy and me that night, because the tube slipped immediately into his trachea instead of his esophagus. We hooked up an oxygen delivery device to the tube, and I began to ventilate him. His skin turned from a frightening shade of blue to deep pink in short order, and he woke up. I then learned that the child had been admitted because of a sore throat and the possible diagnosis of epiglottitis. The disease had shut off his larynx so that he could not breathe, and the lack of oxygen to his brain had caused the seizure. A short time later, his heart would have stopped if we had not intervened. I had been most fortunate to get that tube into his trachea. In those days, the ENT people did not like to leave a tube in the diseased larynx any longer than necessary, so he was immediately scheduled for an emergency tracheostomy. While they were setting up the operating room, I stayed with the child and his family, not wanting anything to happen to the endotracheal tube that was his lifeline for the moment. He was quite awake now and amazingly cooperative. I explained that we would be taking him to the operating room where I would put him to sleep, while the surgeons put a hole in his neck to breathe through so that we could take the tube out of his nose. Although he could not talk because of the tube going between his vocal cords, I could clearly read his lips when he asked, "Am I going to die?" My eyes instantly filled with tears, and with a crack in my voice, I replied, "Not if I can help it, son." He had the tracheostomy, his disease responded quickly to antibiotics, and he went home without further complications.

The point that I wanted to make in relating incidents from my past is that in medicine life-or-death decisions and/or life-or-death actions are daily fare for almost all health care practitioners. I know of no clinical fields in which this is not true. In addition, many of the situations you face will not have been covered specifically in your training, which forces you to think and act quickly based on the principles of diagnosis and treatment you have learned. It will require your utmost diligence throughout your career to conquer the challenges and live up to the expectations of your patients. This is true of all health care professionals, and nurses and paramedics will frequently be asked to hold the line until advanced help arrives on the scene.

There are other points to be learned from the incidents I have just related. One is that you are not always in charge. We like to think that we command a certain amount of omnipotence and can conquer all challenges. We are taught this in popular culture in subtle and not-so-subtle ways. Have there been any movies in which James Bond absolutely loses? Do the doctors on TV series routinely turn disasters into miracles and triumphs? Do the X-Men always conquer evil? Unfortunately, the impossible is not always possible, as in the cases of the child who died in the dryer, the children who died with destroyed livers, and the poor woman who survived a Nazi concentration camp only to die of metastatic cancer of the breast. Realizing that you are not always in charge and cannot always perform miracles is part of the growing-up process in medicine, often an overwhelming and painful experience. Sometimes it is hard to stand back from a tragic situation and realize that you are not responsible, and that the tragedy is not of your making and not yours to bear. You have to maintain your objectivity and recognize that bad things happen to good people, a part of living over which you have no control. Nevertheless, it is humbling and frustrating when you have done your utmost to realize that it was not good enough. Understanding why such tragedies occur is the purview of theology, not medicine.

Another point to learn is that it takes time to become competent to handle the terrible situations you will face. Medical education is in many ways a slow, apprentice-style learning, where responsibility is carefully graded and given to you little by little with increasing degrees of difficulty in decision-making and action. In a proper training program, you will have good supervision and backup until you are finally ready to handle complex problems on your own. Medical education is an ongoing, lifelong process. When you quit learning, you should quit practicing.

Medicine requires a tremendous amount of scientific knowledge, ability, and hard work as well as the capacity to ignore your emotions and to act when you are needed, even in the face of the most repugnant situations. Many times this is not simple; and as I have already said, at some point, you have to let your knowledge, experience, and reflexes go to work for you, letting your emotions surface later over coffee and conversation. In fact, discussing terribly difficult cases with your colleagues in a relaxed setting is more important than you can imagine and should be routinely done in a good practice, both for your own good in releasing all the emotions involved and for the educational benefit of your colleagues. The military calls this debriefing, and it is an important process.

If you have been accepted to medical school, nursing school, or another health care training facility, it is almost certain that you have the capability to do what you will need to do in your practice, but it will take a tremendous amount of work on your part. All one can ask is that you continuously apply yourself to your utmost, learn everything that you can, listen to your mentors, never forget your humanity, remember your goals, and always be grateful that you have an opportunity to help a fellow human being.

I hope this chapter has given you a look at the realities of practicing medicine. These experiences will not be repeated in all specialties, of course; but there are plenty of tragic, dramatic, and unexpected cases awaiting you no matter which road you choose to travel in medicine. It is important that you consider this before you embark on a career to serve those who suffer from an incredible variety of diseases and trauma.

I do not want to leave you feeling that everything in medicine is solemn, serious, and tragic. Sometimes really humorous things happen. One of my favorite stories comes from an obstetrician I worked with years ago. He did his residency training in a hospital in Los Angeles, and one day, he was called to the admitting desk on an urgent basis. When he got there, he found a woman in the late stages of labor sitting in a wheelchair, and he realized that he needed to get her to the delivery suite immediately. They got into the elevator; and about halfway up, she delivered the baby, upon which she began to cry despondently about delivering in an elevator. My friend told her not to feel badly because a year ago, a woman had actually delivered on the front lawn of the hospital. Sobbing even louder, she replied, "I know! That was me!"

One day, I was inducing anesthesia in an eight-year-old boy who was going to have an ENT procedure. He was extraordinarily cooperative, and I was doing a slow, careful induction by gradually increasing the concentration of anesthetic gas flowing into the mask over his face. To distract him, I talked about the Saturday morning cartoons I watched with my kids and then began to talk about my kids' favorite breakfast cereals. Suddenly, he reached up, moved the mask away from his face a little, and said to me very clearly, "I think if you'd shut up, I could fall asleep!" The nursing staff burst into laughter and made certain that I never forgot that one.

*An autobiography usually reveals nothing bad
about its writer except his memory.*
—Franklin P. Jones

Chapter 3

Who Am I?

Now that you have already read a little bit about what I have done, perhaps you might wish to learn a little bit more about me and from where I've come. I had not really considered this book as an autobiography, but it has turned out that way to a degree; just the same, it is important for me to offer you some of my history so that you have an idea as to what makes me tick before I offer you my opinions or anything else. Of course, if you do not care about who I am, just skip this chapter and go on to the next. I threw this stuff in at no extra charge anyway, and not reading it will not ruin the rest.

I am descended on my father's side from an early settler in Stonington, Connecticut, named Edmund Fanning, who fled from Limerick, Ireland, in 1653 to escape the horrors of Oliver Cromwell's army that was ravaging the country in those days. We have a two-volume book about the descendants of Edmund written in the 1920s; and my grandfather, who was born in Geneseo, New York, is listed in one of the last generations of the book. My paternal grandmother was from Minto, a tiny town in southern Scotland near Jedburgh. My mother's father was born in Pennsylvania, a descendant of English settlers. Her mother was the daughter of Swedish immigrants. I haven't a clue as to how any of these people met and fell in love. No one in the family was highly educated, except for a relative of my grandmother Fanning who was a noted preacher in Scotland.

My father left school in his early teens to go to work to help support his large family. A highly intelligent man, he did well at work and ultimately took night school courses at the Rochester Institute of Technology in Rochester, New York, to supplement his meager formal education. Mother never finished high school. I have no idea of how she and my father met or how long they dated. They never talked about it. She married my father when she was twenty years old, and I came along about ten months later.

I was born in Rochester, New York, in the summer of 1940, destined to be my parents' only child. Dad worked for Taylor Instrument Co., an institution that produced instruments that controlled a variety of industrial processes and also produced consumer products, such as thermometers, barometers, and sphygmomanometers. He worked for them over fifty years. I remember little of my early life, save that we lived on a street called English Road in a near northwestern suburb of Rochester called Greece in a lower middle-class neighborhood. My father worked dreadfully long hours during World War II. Although we didn't know why then, in later years, we learned that his work involved something quite secret on an extremely hush-hush undertaking known as the "Manhattan Project." I have no idea what his role was, but he showed me the lapel pin he received from the government acknowledging his participation.

In January 1946, my father was promoted and transferred to Tulsa, Oklahoma. Our household goods were packed onto a big green and yellow truck with a picture of an old sailing ship and the word "Mayflower" on the side. As we had no car during the war, we took the train to Tulsa, a trip I do not remember in the least. I do remember our first days in Tulsa and meeting Bobby Davis who would be my best friend during the seven years we lived there. He was one year ahead of me in school and lived just three doors down the street. During those seven years, he and I played the roles of every cowboy and soldier who ever lived as well as building tanks on our wagons and a laboratory to study worms in the crawl space under his house. Bobby had an enormous, wild imagination, so we never lacked for things to do. If we had some cardboard and a few pieces of wood, we would try to build something.

We ran around the neighborhood gleefully playing our games with no regard for property lines or fences and with our voices at full blast most of the time. One of my favorite stories involves a conversation my mother had with our next-door neighbor. He was telling her that he could not stand Bobby Davis. She assured him that this was not uncommon, that one could often tolerate things in one's own kids but be vexed by similar traits or activities in others' children. He thought for a moment and then shook his head affirmatively. "You're right," he said, "I can't stand Gary either!"

During first grade, I felt sick one morning and did not want to go to school, something unusual for me. I had a fever, so my mother called the doctor. When he came, he examined me and apparently heard a heart murmur for he announced to my mother that he suspected that I had contracted rheumatic fever, a condition affecting the valves of my heart. The treatment was strict bed rest and little else. There was not much penicillin available to the general public in January 1947, and I think it was just starting to be used for that diagnosis in any case. So for three months, I lay in bed with nothing to do but color, read, listen to a radio, try to do schoolwork sent home to me, and eat. My mother even carried me to the bathroom, just a few feet from my bedroom in the small house in which we lived.

I'll interrupt myself long enough to say how wonderful I used to feel when the doctor came to our house when I was sick. There was magic in his black bag, his thermometer, his stethoscope, and even in the rustling sound his shirtsleeve made within his coat sleeve when he examined me. Once a doctor came and, to examine my pharynx, he got up on the bed and straddled me to shove a teaspoon into my mouth and down my throat. Mercifully, my mother never called that son of a bitch again. House calls are nearly gone. Scientific medical practice is much improved, but the magic of the doctor in your bedroom was magnificent.

Once a week, we had to go to the doctor's office for a blood test. Mom called a taxi for the trip, as we still had no car. The most frequent cab driver to respond to the call was a jolly black man with a huge belly. My mother used to tease him about it, because he could hardly fit behind the wheel. He would laugh good-naturedly at her teasing and razz her in return. I always looked forward to seeing him and liked him a lot. He was very kind to Mom and me. The laws of Oklahoma in those days included strict segregation. There were black and white drinking fountains, black and white restrooms, and separate housing areas. I hated that discrimination, not only because of what I observed but also because my parents hated it and spoke quite openly against it. It was a cruel and completely unjustified practice, and I am most happy it is gone.

When the three months was over, I had gained twenty-five pounds and could hardly walk I was so weak. I was not allowed to run, was limited in my gym activities, and became extremely winded with only moderate physical activity. As a result of this, I never really liked vigorous exercise, especially running, and never developed any athletic prowess; however, it did not make me short of breath to read and study, so I became an avid student. Years later, I was able to exercise normally and enjoyed physical activity, but never with the zeal I might have enjoyed without that three-month imprisonment in bed.

I started going to church when we lived in Tulsa. My parents were not particularly religious, so I got myself up on Sunday morning and walked to the Baptist church not far from where we lived. My first Sunday school teacher was a man named Mr. Sebastian, a wonderful storyteller and a true believer, who filled us in on the basic tenets of the faith. After Sunday school, we were invited to attend the regular church service, which I did. The preacher was typical of most Southern Baptist ministers of the day in that he was charismatic, demonstrative, loud, and filled with warnings of hellfire and brimstone for the unfaithful. Abe Lincoln said, "When I hear a man preach, I like to see him act as if he were fighting bees." Abe would have liked this man. He often preached on the evils of smoking and drinking, both of which my parents were clearly guilty, leaving me to worry about their salvation. This was also the source of my first real lesson in hypocrisy. One Saturday, Bobby Davis and I had just come out of the local movie theater and were headed for the nearby dime store to invest the five or ten cents left over from our movie money. As we turned a corner, I saw the choirmaster of our church coming toward us lighting up a cigarette. Lordy, lordy, lordy! It shook me to the core to see this man smoking after all the warnings we had heard each Sunday morning from the pulpit of our church where he sat and shouted amen to the preacher's rants. I wish that this had been the only example of hypocrisy encountered in my lifetime. It certainly was one of the least important.

In the summer of 1952, my father received another promotion, one that required us to return to Rochester for him to assume his new position in the home factory. My parents were a bit sad about leaving Tulsa, but I was excited because of all the stories I had heard from my parents, and because most of my relatives were in the Rochester area. I remember the three-day road trip quite well. I especially enjoyed watching television in our motel rooms, because my father didn't want one of the "damn things" in our house. In our 1941 De Soto, we drove from Tulsa through Missouri, Illinois, Indiana, Ohio, Pennsylvania, and finally to New York. Indiana had one of the first four-lane divided highways, and you were allowed to drive the breakneck speed of fifty-five miles per hour. I distinctly remember reading the Burma Shave signs as we drove along. It is too bad that they have disappeared, as they were funny and entertaining. You will find a nice collection of them at the House on the Rock near Spring Green, Wisconsin.

When we got to Rochester, we stayed with my aunt, uncle, and cousin while my parents searched for a house. After a long search, they finally found one in a little town west of Rochester called Spencerport. Having accompanied my parents in their search for a house, my aunt and uncle found a house in Spencerport that they liked and decided to move there too. As a result, my cousin Lee and I started Spencerport Central School together, although he was one year ahead of me.

Spencerport was a super town in which to grow up in the 1950s. Its population was about 3,200, and it was located right on the Barge Canal, the modern successor of the old Erie Canal, some of which was still there if you knew where to look. It had a quaint main street, friendly people, neat and clean neighborhoods, and a rustic, rural quality that excited me. It was a safe place for kids, and you could walk or ride your bike everywhere. The school was also super. The teachers, for the most part, were excellent, helpful, and caring. Lee and I instantly felt at home in school and quickly made friends. I felt fortunate then, and feel so now, that my parents chose to settle in this little burg.

Life was good in Spencerport. I enjoyed many activities in addition to wonderful outdoor recreation, such as swimming, biking, fishing, and hunting. I joined the local drum and bugle corps early on, and this led to my joining the high school band, where I played trumpet for the first two years and baritone sax for the last two. I have mentioned that we had good teachers in our little school, but two of them stand out as the best I ever knew. The first, John Betlem, was my English teacher freshman and sophomore years. I had him as a study hall teacher in junior high and was scared to death of him; but in English class, he was amazing. Never had I learned so much and had so much fun at the same time. He was charismatic, funny, and smart. He helped us through the drudgery of learning the parts of speech and of parsing sentences. He rewarded us by introducing us to literature and by telling us wonderful stories. Two impressive placards hung on the wall in his room. One, right beneath the clock, read, "Time passes, will you?" The second, not far away, mysteriously read, "Good mother is bad mother for me." We all chewed on that one for a while until we finally caught its meaning. The second excellent teacher was Ralph Jordan, our math teacher. Ralph always treated us as adults, and in return, he received the respect and attention that he showed us. His mind was incredible. It was so much fun to watch him ponder a difficult math problem and then share his musings with us as he wrote the equations on the blackboard. He was prone to lean against that board, and his suits were chronically covered with chalk dust on the back. High school was a fun time.

A few weeks before turning sixteen, I got a part-time job with an electrician who lived just down the street from us. His name was Ansel Jones Brennan, an unforgettable character who was exceptionally kind and generous to me. We did mostly residential wiring, but we did some commercial work too. It was a fun job that required careful thinking as well as a lot of physical labor. It was much preferable to the job in the grocery store I had held for two years. I worked for Ansel after school and on Saturday in high school and full-time in the summer and on school breaks during my college years. In addition to learning something about the electrical trade, I also learned that for me, a pursuit in life that depended more on brains than on brawn was something desirable and worth working hard to achieve.

The best part of living in Spencerport was that it was there I met my beloved, Arline Hammar. We were both sixteen, she in her senior year and I in my junior. She had skipped a grade by doing two grades in one year at the one-room elementary school she had attended. I got up the courage to ask her to go on a hayride, and she said she would ask her parents for permission. Her mother was about to say no when her father spoke up and said yes. He was ever my favorite after that. We double-dated on the hayride with Chip Evans and his date. Chip was a good friend and was just slightly older, so he was able to drive a car at night. He was a clean, dependable lad, the kind of fellow you would pick as a friend for your own children. We had a lot of fun on that hayride, and though Arline and I had known each other for a long time, it was really a case of love at first date. We never looked back after that night of October 10, 1956, and we have been faithfully in love ever since.

After high school, Arline went to Russell Sage College in Troy, New York; and a year later, I went to Hamilton College in Clinton, New York. It was and still is an excellent institution, but I cannot honestly say that I really enjoyed college. There were simply two things on my mind: Arline and medical school. Arline and I did not see much of each other during our college years, and despite having good friends and a lot of schoolwork, I lived in a perpetual state of loneliness. I hung out with my two best friends, both of whom were also premed students. Thank God for their friendship, but I still missed Arline terribly. We did not have cars, there was no e-mail, there were no cell phones or texting, and landline phone calls were expensive. The glue that held us together was our daily letter writing. When you write to a person every day and receive a letter in return, you get to know a lot about that person and about yourself. To everyone's surprise, our romance stayed hot; and thanks in no small part to our devotion to each other then, it still is.

Arline and I were married the summer I graduated from college. Having graduated a year earlier, she taught school during the year before we were married, living with her parents and saving as much as she could. We were married in the White Church (congregational) in Spencerport, the church that we attended during our teens and where we were both baptized. When we returned from our honeymoon, we moved to Syracuse, where I started medical school and she taught school.

The four years of medical school were among the happiest of our lives. We had nothing but each other, hard work, and hope; but we took advantage of enjoying each other's company as much as we could to make up for the previous five years of loneliness. Being a teacher, she was no less strict with the student living in our apartment than she was with those attending her classes. I studied diligently, and she helped in every way that she could, including helping me studying the life cycles of parasites and other rote memorization tasks. I loved medical school, and the four years went faster than I could ever imagine. I studied hard, held a part-time job during my junior and senior years, and enjoyed my limited free time with my beautiful bride. Studying the medical sciences in the first two years was interesting and challenging, but the real delight came in the last two years as we went through our clinical rotations. Learning to interact with patients and observing the disease entities we had read about in books was wonderful. My part-time job as an extern at St. Joseph Hospital exposed me to even more clinical pathology and gave me the opportunity to deal with patients in a way similar to what I would be doing as an intern when I graduated. All in all, medical school for me was everything that college had not been.

I was matched to the University of Rochester's Strong Memorial Hospital for a straight surgical internship. It was a terribly difficult year. The work itself was not so hard, although it was quite demanding. It was the time commitment that was so tough: thirty-six hours on duty and twelve hours off (if you were lucky). We all got precious little sleep, a commodity considered a luxury for mere interns. Once again, Arline and I hardly saw each other that year. She was fortunate to get a teaching job in the school in which she had taught the year before we were married.

On the first day of internship, Dr. Charles Rob, chief of surgery, told us that this would be a clinical year, and that we would not have much time for reading. He was spot-on in that assessment. We did not have time to do anything but work. Everyone seemed to be afraid of Dr. Rob. He had reportedly fired a resident some years earlier, so nobody wanted to make any mistakes and incur his wrath. I was not interested in becoming a general surgeon and thus had less fear, but I always tried to do my best. I grew fond of Dr. Rob and learned a great deal from him during the four years I knew him. In addition to being an excellent surgeon and a highly respected academician, he was a true physician who treated his patients with love, respect, and utmost skill. The month I spent on his service was one of the hardest and best of my year. It was hardest because of the two residents assigned to his service who did not want me to screw up and reflect badly on them, and best because I learned so much from Dr. Rob.

During my internship year, life took an unexpected twist. Each of us was subject to military duty after completing an internship. A few got away without being drafted, but those who had received deferments to finish college and medical school, as I had, were inescapably in the crosshairs of the draft boards. I applied to something called the Berry Plan along with virtually everyone I knew. If you were accepted into this plan, you were deferred to finish the specialty training for which you had applied before going on active duty. I had applied for deferment to train in ENT, but I was not accepted. If you were not accepted, you could choose to enter the service immediately after internship or after one additional year of training. As I was required to do a year of general surgical residency before entering an ENT training program, I took the additional year option.

About halfway through my internship, I began to question the wisdom of my becoming an ENT surgeon after all. I got curious as to what was happening on the other side of the ether screen and started talking to the anesthesiologists. It also dawned on me that the best part of the day for me was the time in the operating room. I liked the environment, the people, and the excitement. I suddenly concluded that the only physician who spends virtually all day in the operating room is the anesthesiologist. As I thought about it and talked about it with Arline, the more I became convinced that this was what I should do. I went to Alastair Gillies, chairman of the Department of Anesthesiology, and talked with him about my feelings. He was delighted and offered me a residency on the spot. I accepted immediately and have never once regretted my decision. The U.S. Army liked it too, because when I informed them that I was going to use my year after internship to train in anesthesiology, they wrote back and told me to stay until I had completed my full training in that discipline.

If internship had been a year of hell, residency was three years of heaven. I felt like I was learning something new every day, and the attending physicians were superb teachers. I was thoroughly impressed that the professor and chairman himself guided me through the anesthetics on my first day of residency, which was a Saturday. I still remember Alastair's advice to me on that beginning day: "Gary, always help the surgeons all you can, because they need all the help they can get." I can honestly say that I have tried hard to live up to that advice. During my last two years of residency, I was fortunate to do research with a wonderful man named Frank Colgan. Frank was smart, laid back, friendly, and innovative. He wore a perpetual smile and kept his brain hot with ideas like some people keep a pot of coffee brewing all day long. We did research in the area of pulmonary physiology, and the things I learned working with Frank helped me during my entire career. Although doing research with Frank was a lot of fun and highly rewarding with regard to knowledge gained, I wanted to be a clinician more than anything else. Taking care of patients was my real desire, and that is where I ultimately landed. I have not regretted that, despite what I might have missed.

While in residency, Arline and I had our first two children, Michael and Mary Ellen. They were exactly two years apart, and we took to the job of parenting remarkably well. As Arline and I had been only children, we were determined to have more than one, and I am glad that we were so blessed. About two months before the end of residency, Arline discovered that we were going to have a third. It was a wonderful surprise, to say the least, and we still consider our children as our most important blessings in life.

After residency, I spent two years in the U.S. Army, where I was stationed at Fort Knox, Kentucky. After being there for only a month, I was named chief of anesthesia and operative services, a position for which I hardly felt qualified. A few months later, another anesthesiologist with more time in rank came back from Vietnam and assumed that position. He and I were good friends and got along well with each other and with the other members of the department. The nurse anesthetists we worked with were superb. It was a busy hospital, and we did about everything except heart surgery and neurosurgery. Our third child, Sarah, was born there in January 1971, a wonderful gift for her mother and me. I really enjoyed my experience as a physician in the army. We were a large group of young physicians newly out of training, and we got along just fine. It was a good two years. I am honored to have served the soldiers who fought in Vietnam and their families.

From Fort Knox, Kentucky, we moved to Iowa in July 1972, where I joined a large multispecialty group in a small university city. The way in which we ended up in Iowa tells a lot about Arline and me. Toward the end of my residency, we began to explore seriously where we might want to settle after getting out of the army. We contemplated moving to the west coast because we wanted to get away from the east coast. One day, I looked at a population density map of the United States and realized that the country looks just like a set of parentheses on one of these charts, because the densest population is along both coasts. This started us thinking about the interior of the country where things looked a bit less crowded. One Sunday, there was an article in our local paper about a troop of boy scouts burning fields of wild marijuana plants in Iowa. Hemp had been grown in Iowa during the war for rope and burlap and had gone wild. The reporter interviewed the scoutmaster who said that he was just trying to make a point with the boys that marijuana is merely a weed and not something worth saving, buying, or dying over. The reporter then went to the Haight-Ashbury section of San Francisco and interviewed a hippie. He told him that boy scouts were burning marijuana in Iowa and asked if he wanted to go up there and get some before they destroyed it all.

The hippie replied, "No man, that grass ain't no good. The best grass grows in Mexico, not Iowa. Besides, who'd want to go to Iowa?"

Right away upon reading that, we figured that Iowa must be a pretty nice place. If it was not attractive to hippies, it certainly was attractive to us. I began looking for opportunities in Iowa and learned of a multispecialty clinic that happened to be known to some colleagues in Rochester whom I trusted a lot. During my first year in the army, Arline and I took a quick trip there and were quite impressed with both the town and the clinic. I was offered a position to begin when I finished my service, and I accepted.

Being in practice at last and having our first house was so exciting for us after all those years of work and sacrifice. We loved our new home and our new community. It was and still is a magnificent small city, and the clinic is an exceptionally fine medical institution for a city of any size. It turned out to be a safe, pleasant place to live and raise children, and the clinic was a perfect place to practice. All the physicians had been well trained, and the atmosphere felt to a large extent like an academic one. We had made a good choice.

In December 1972, one of the senior surgeons asked me if I would be interested in assuming the position of medical director of the emergency medical system (EMS) squad that was just forming. The hospital had received some federal money to buy a new ambulance and we needed to train emergency medical technicians (EMTs) for its use. The Department of Transportation in those days had produced a modular course for the training of EMTs, and my first job was to coordinate the course and find lecturers among my colleagues to teach the various modules. We had a superb group of young people for our first students and EMT employees. After their basic training, we slowly increased their abilities and responsibilities, first teaching them by extensive hands-on training to start IVs and ultimately to do things like endotracheal intubation and finally defibrillation. The medical staff assumed a large liability risk in allowing this, because there was no law at this time governing the practice of paramedics. As the procedures we were allowing them to perform were clearly in the realm of the practice of medicine, we worried that they might be guilty of practicing medicine without a license. This same situation was occurring nationwide at the time, and eventually a movement took root that led to the development of paramedic laws and certification in many states. I was honored to be on the ad hoc committee appointed by Gov. Bob Ray to write the paramedic law in Iowa, and our hospital had the first fully approved paramedic unit in the state. Our paramedics easily passed the state examination for certification, and two of them held certificates #1 and #2. I am very proud of my association with the paramedics at that institution, and I consider my work with them to be the most significant contribution to patient care of my career. Many of those first paramedics have gone on to great careers in high places, and I am honored to have been part of their lives.

We became Episcopalians while living in Iowa. We went to a service at the Episcopal church, did a lot of reading about the faith, and decided we would join. One afternoon, I called the rector of the Episcopal parish, Fr. Paul Goodland, and asked if I could talk to him sometime about becoming an Episcopalian. His immediate answer was, "What are you doing right now?" That was the attitude I was looking for, and he and I became good friends. Choosing to attend that church was one of the best decisions we ever made, for we became friends with a whole group of wonderful people.

Paul Goodland was a unique human being, devout, practical, and tough. He was mayor of our city for two terms, and his motto was, "Fair in all things, neutral in none." His card listed several local restaurants along with the days of the week he would be having breakfast in each. People could meet him there and discuss anything they wished. I never heard him waffle an answer just to make someone like him. He treated everyone with love and respect, but he never backed down in an argument. He and his wife, Sally, retired just at the same time we left Iowa. We kept in touch with them until they both passed away. I still miss his unexpected phone calls asking me some question related to medicine. He never said hello, choosing simply to start the conversation and expecting you to recognize his voice, which I always did.

After nearly twenty years of practicing medicine and raising our children in Iowa, I grew restless and decided I might want to consider another practice. A large part of my restlessness came from the fact that I was taking so much call. I finally decided that if an opportunity came along in an outpatient setting, I would look at it. One day, I received a circular in the mail describing a position for an anesthesiologist in northern Illinois in a freestanding surgery center devoted to ophthalmology. It was called the Hauser-Ross Eye Institute, named for Lynn Hauser and her husband Neil Ross, the owners of the practice. I visited them twice and was so impressed with them and their entire staff that I accepted the job offer.

We left Iowa in August 1991, leaving the beautiful house we had built in 1979 in forty acres of woods. Working at the Hauser-Ross Eye Institute was terrific for me from the outset. Lynn and Neil were superb surgeons and ran the institution like a benevolent queen and king, and the surgery center was an unusually pleasant place to work. The only thing I missed was my daily interaction with my anesthesia colleagues in Iowa. I was initially taught to do eye blocks by a certified registered nurse anesthetist (CRNA), who left about a month after I arrived. Another CRNA was there who monitored the patients in the OR while I did the blocks in the preoperative area, and we worked closely together when we did general anesthetics. His name was Larry Larson, and he and I got along better than brothers. We both liked golf, good food, and reading about World War II. He had a great sense of humor and was wonderful to our patients. I missed him terribly when he retired and even more when he passed away. I enjoyed working with the exceptionally fine surgeons at the institute and learned that helping in ophthalmic surgery could be challenging, rewarding, and fun. The nurses and support staff at Hauser-Ross were excellent. They were helpful to me, and they treated our patients with love, compassion, and skill. When I finally retired, leaving them was undoubtedly the toughest part.

Lynn Hauser and Neil Ross made my employment conditional on two things: attending a meeting of the Ophthalmic Anesthesia Society (OAS) and spending a day with Robert Hustead, MD, in Wichita, Kansas. Bob was an ophthalmic anesthesiologist and founder of OAS. Both experiences were invaluable to me, and I quickly became active in the society. Early in my new practice, Lynn and Neil brought Bob Hustead and Roy Hamilton, an ophthalmic anesthesiologist who practiced in Calgary, Alberta, Canada, to

Sycamore to consult with me and give me pointers. We ultimately dissected an orbit together at Northern Illinois University and presented a tape of the dissection at the next OAS meeting. It was a huge success and started me on my way in the society. I was ultimately elected for a term as president and served about seven years as the planner of the annual meeting, as well as editor of the newsletter. This all resulted in my being asked to come to England to lecture about anatomy and block technique and to serve as a curbside consultant for the anesthesiologists there as they organized their own British Ophthalmic Anaesthesia Society. A few years later, after a couple of trips to England, two of the British anesthesiologists, Chandra Kumar and Chris Dodds, asked me to work with them to edit and write a textbook of ophthalmic anesthesia, which I did. The book—*Ophthalmic Anaesthesia* by Kumar, Dodds, and Fanning (Swets & Zeitlinger, Lisse, the Netherlands, 2002)—got good reviews and was popular in the field. Without having joined the Hauser-Ross Eye Institute, none of this would have happened; and I would have missed an important, rewarding, and enriching part of my life.

We attended a small church in De Kalb when we lived in Illinois, the Church of St. Paul, Episcopal. It was much smaller than the one in Iowa, but the people were equally wonderful. We made friends there quickly and became extremely active in the church. Arline had served on the vestry in Iowa, and I served on it at St. Paul's. Arline had also been the head of the Altar Guild in Iowa and quickly was welcomed into a similar role in De Kalb. We certainly enjoyed our association with this church and its people.

I retired from the Hauser-Ross Eye Institute in August 2007, and we moved to a suburb of St. Paul to be closer to both of our daughters and to our three grandchildren, Evelyn, Alex, and John, who live in the Twin Cities area. We have loved being here and being near them. We all attend the same church, a friendly Episcopal church in Edina called St. Albans. The priest, Fr. John Peters, gives the best sermons I have ever heard.

I did not stay fully retired for long. Old friends in Madison, Wisconsin, whom I had met through OAS, asked me to work there for a few months while they hired and trained a new person. Arline and I went there in January 2008, staying in the Residence Inn and returning home to check the mail and our town house about every two weekends. I immediately enjoyed working at the Davis Duehr Dean Eye Surgery Center in Madison and have been treated with great kindness by everyone there. The surgeons at that institution are superb, and working with them is incredibly pleasant. They epitomize everything good that I will have to say about doctors in the rest of this book. The nursing and support staff are also wonderful and have made me part of their family. We ended up being there for eight months before slipping back into retirement. I still go there about twelve to sixteen weeks a year to fill in for Joan McGrath and Neal Janquart when they take well-earned vacations or go to meetings. Thus, I have a sweet deal: enjoying retirement, still getting to do what I love, and working with people who are exceptionally skilled, dedicated, and congenial.

That brings us up to date. You now know more about me than you no doubt wanted to know, but perhaps it will help you understand my perspective when I start barking orders and giving you opinions. It has not been an exceptional life by any means, but I have enjoyed it and tried to do my best. There is a lot more to tell than I have related in this chapter, of course, but you will find plenty of vignettes scattered throughout the remainder of the book to expand upon what I have said here, assuming, of course, that you are brave enough to read more.

One who maintains cleanliness keeps away diseases.
—Sam Veda

Chapter 4

Wash Your Hands

I told you that I would be giving you advice, and none is more basic than this: *wash your hands*! It seems like a simple command; nonetheless, too many people forget this most fundamental of disease-prevention techniques. It should not surprise you that all health care professionals can spread disease and were guilty of doing so on a wholesale basis in the past. It can still happen, of course. Hands are busy things that touch multiple items in the course of a day. For us, that means touching multiple patients, some of whom are infected with dangerous organisms that can easily and unknowingly be transmitted to other human beings. Hopefully, we all wear disposable gloves most of the time now and routinely change them between patients, but it serves us well to remember our history and to revere those who first advised us to wash our hands. Our duty is to first do no harm, and the cornerstone of that duty is cleanliness.

You probably do not know the name Ignaz Semmelweis. You should. Look him up on Wikipedia if you don't know his story. Better yet, read the novel, *The Cry and the Covenant* by Morton Thompson (Doubleday & Co.), a romanticized version of Semmelweis's life first published in 1949. You can still get a used paperback copy of it (Buccaneer Books Inc.) through Amazon.com. The book should be required reading for all medical and nursing students and students of all the allied health fields, but, unfortunately, it is not.

Ignaz Semmelweis was born in Hungary in 1818. He became a physician specializing in obstetrics and obtained a position at a hospital in Vienna. In those days, Austrians considered Hungarians as second-class (or worse) citizens and treated them badly. In addition, he was Jewish, which lowered his status even more in those days. Puerperal fever, a highly fatal disease, was rampant in the hospitals of Europe in the mid-nineteenth century, and no one knew the cause. Women begged to deliver at home rather than taking a chance of dying in the hospital. We now recognize puerperal fever as a bacterial disease, usually streptococcal, of the lining of the uterus (endometrium) following delivery. At that time, however, the germ theory of disease, as later proven by Pasteur, had yet to be fully proposed and confirmed. Ignaz Semmelweis observed that the incidence of death from the disease was much higher in the clinic attended by physicians than in the clinic attended by midwives. He also had a friend who died after cutting himself accidentally with a scalpel while doing an autopsy on a woman who had died of puerperal fever. The symptoms of his dying friend reminded Ignaz of puerperal fever, leading him to the conclusion that something had been transferred to his friend from the dead woman by the scalpel. He further concluded that perhaps the physicians in the clinic with the high death rate were somehow responsible for spreading some unknown agent from patient to patient.

Doctors in those times were proud of their bloodstained coats and dirty hands, symbols of their diligence and success. In his own ward, Semmelweis insisted that the medical staff wash their hands between patients in a solution of chlorinated lime. Despite the fact that he demonstrated a remarkable drop in the incidence of death from puerperal fever, he was laughed at and scorned by his colleagues. He continued to show remarkable results despite this derision, but his pleas for others to copy his practice went largely unheeded. He ultimately went insane and actually died of septicemia himself. The works of Pasteur and finally of Joseph Lister ultimately vindicated Semmelweis's findings and at last ushered in the era of antiseptic surgery. It is sad that Semmelweis is all but forgotten; nonetheless, his insights and bravery deserve remembering. Whenever you wash your hands, say, "Thank you, Ignaz!"

There are several lessons to be learned from the story of Ignaz Semmelweis. First of all, we should pay homage to those who went before us and made monumental discoveries for the good of mankind. I read *The Cry and the Covenant* before entering medical school; and to this very day, I think of Ignaz Semmelweis when I wash my hands, which I do frequently. Second, everyone is capable of making an observation and putting two and two together. A good example is that of Edward Jenner, who observed that milkmaids who contracted cowpox never suffered from smallpox, which led him to begin the practice of vaccination, a simple procedure that has saved countless lives; in fact, hand washing and vaccination have collectively saved more lives than all the surgery ever performed. Unfortunately, many of us are unreceptive to new ideas, our own or others, especially when we are being educated (indoctrinated?) by those older and presumably wiser than us. Some of us are so entrenched in our ways that we simply ignore anything new. Observation is the origin of discovery, and if what we observe in good scientific fashion does not exactly agree with what we have been taught, we ought to question what we have been taught.

Third, we need to listen when someone has a new idea, especially if that idea has been subjected to the rigors of scientific reasoning. I hope that they taught you about the scientific method in college, and that you took to heart what they taught you, because you will be using the tenets of the scientific method throughout your career.

Fourth, listen to the message intensely and do not pay so much attention to the messenger. If Ignaz Semmelweis had been Austrian instead of Hungarian, they might have listened to him and thousands of lives might have been saved. The intense bigotry of the nineteenth century had cost thousands of women their lives because narrow-minded Austrian physicians would not listen to the wise counsel of a Hungarian colleague, especially a Jewish one. You will hear me say it again: Bigotry has no place in medicine (or anywhere else, for that matter).

An infectious disease specialist who was the most boring speaker I ever heard gave the first lecture I attended on the subject of HIV. His slides were black with white lettering and little bitty print and were filled with unreadable numbers and statistics. Despite his drone and terrible visual aids, the information he was giving us was both fascinating and important. Remember that the message transcends the messenger. A corollary is that the slick, handsome, charismatic lecturer may grab your attention, but beware that his material may be little better than worthless. Always listen with a critical ear and an open mind. You never know from where an exceptionally good idea or discovery will come, and you never know when it will come. Just be sure that you are in a receptive mood when it does.

In cataract surgery, the pressure inside the eye can be problematic for the surgeon, and it sometimes goes up during the procedure. Classically, surgeons ask for the patient to be given something called mannitol, a high molecular weight sugar that acts osmotically to draw fluid out of the eye. Unfortunately, it draws fluid out of other tissues as well, delivering it to the kidneys via the circulatory system and hence to the bladder. So we end up with a patient whom we want to lie quite still but who now has a bladder full of urine and is writhing in discomfort while undergoing a delicate procedure under local anesthesia. This is not a good situation, to be sure.

As a speaker attending a medical meeting in England, I was fortunate to attend a dinner and cocktail party hosted by Robert and Ursula Johnson. Bob is an anesthesiologist and was in charge of the meeting. In addition, they are friends who have visited Arline and me when we lived in Sycamore, and we still keep in touch. Over a glass of wine, I had a delightful conversation with a knowledgeable and congenial anesthesiologist from Mumbai, India. He asked me if I had ever tried using intravenous lidocaine (a local anesthetic drug) to reduce the pressure in the eye during cataract surgery. I had not. He informed me that it worked beautifully and asked if he could send me some data that I might want to consider publishing in the newsletter of the Ophthalmic Anesthesia Society. As I was editor of that publication at the time, I said I would be happy to look at his work. He sent me the data, which was quite impressive. I tried his technique in my own practice many times, had marvelous results, and stopped using mannitol. I published his data twice in *OASIS* (the society's newsletter) and have since passed his information on to others at multiple medical meetings. Keep your mind, eyes, and ears open. You never know when there is something important to learn.

Finally, the experience of Ignaz Semmelweis tells you to WASH YOUR HANDS! In addition to doing that, be faithful in wearing gloves routinely and protective clothing when necessary. It is important that you protect your patients from infectious diseases, but it is equally important for you to protect yourself, your family, and the community at large.

Actually, washing your hands is just a start. Physicians and nurses and all allied health personnel should be epitomes of good grooming. A daily routine of bathing (or showering), applying underarm deodorant, and wearing clean clothes is a start. You may think me a simpleton or a grouch for saying these things, but I have seen it all, believe me. A professional should look like a professional, and for a member of the health care profession that means being clean, nonconfrontational, and modest in your dress and pleasant in your appearance. Take the piercings out of your lips, tongue, eyelids, eyebrows, and so forth. They are offensive to many people, me included. A pair of pierced earrings for women may be nice, but they are still not as acceptable for men in our profession. I cannot say much about piercings in places that are not normally seen in polite company (and there are damn few of those left these days!), but I can say you will never find piercings on me. I could say the same about tattoos. I would like my doctor or nurse to look like a doctor or nurse, thank you very much, not like a carnival worker or professional wrestler. Now I see absolutely nothing wrong with carnival workers or professional wrestlers being tattooed, but I would argue that it is inappropriate for health care providers to be so adorned. I once saw a bumper sticker advertising a tattoo parlor that read, "Take Pride in Your Hide!" Take pride that your hide is clean and unadorned. Treat it as the marvelous organ that it is, not like a canvas covered with art. If you have facial hair, be sure that it is neatly and closely trimmed. Hair is dirty, and it will not do to drag a two-foot-long beard across your poor patient while listening to the heart and lungs with your stethoscope. You will be shocked at some of the things you will find in some patients' hair if you examine them carefully. Just be sure that the same cannot be said of yours. You may now think of me as an old fuddy-duddy for this advice and for swimming upstream against popular culture and fashion; however, I can assure you that appearances are still important, especially in certain areas of society including the medical profession. If you want to be regarded and esteemed as a medical professional, dress the part. What people do in other professions and lines of work is their own business, but you should look clean, neat, and never "in your face."

We have reached an age of incredible informality of dress. I am so old that I remember when traveling by air meant wearing a suit and tie. Most good restaurants in those days also required a gentleman to wear a coat and tie. Certain industries still expect their men and women to dress in "business formal" on a day-to-day basis, but the medical profession is less formal than it once was. As a result, it is often hard to tell who's who in the hospital or clinic setting these days. It is unlikely that our society will return to the more rigid dress codes of a few years past; even so, it is important to be clean and well groomed, albeit less formally so. The last thing that people who are sick want to see is someone leaning over them with a stethoscope who looks as though he or she just climbed out of a gravel pit or walked in out of the barn after doing a little strategic shoveling. Be careful that you do not wear good-looking clothing that is infrequently cleaned, such as suits and ties, because cleanliness is way more important than looking like a banker. Blue jeans are certainly not appropriate daily wear save in some rural settings where they might be quite acceptable so long as they are clean. They might be appropriate on weekends in other locales when you are on call and working in the yard or garage or attending one of your children's sporting events. In England, they discourage the wearing of ties because they are infrequently, if ever, cleaned. A clean, starched white (or any color) coat that is frequently and thoroughly laundered makes a good impression and is certainly acceptable by all. If you have to see a patient who is suffering a dangerous infectious disease, remove the white coat and put on appropriate barrier clothing, gloves, and facemask before entering the patient's room.

I can hear my critics already: "Fanning doesn't approve of piercings, tattoos, blue jeans, facial hair, or anything else modern and fashionable!" That may be a fair assessment after reading all the above, but it is only partially true. I disapprove of those things *for physicians and health care personnel.* You must get used to the fact that the majority of our patients have high expectations of us in many areas, including our appearance. They expect the same of lawyers, clergy, bankers, and others. I am not a judge and would not condemn somebody for having a tattoo or a pierced eyebrow, even if either offended me personally, which they sometimes do. I am really repulsed by a waiter, waitress, or clerk whose face is covered with piercings and whose visible skin is covered with weird and occasionally lewd tattoos. Being offended by such things is my own hang-up, I freely admit, so knock off the Bronx cheers. I probably offend them because of the way I look. Touché. Keep in mind that I would be willing to take up arms against a government that would seek to ban such things as piercings and tattoos. Personal freedom is important to us all, and we should have the right to practice it so long as the practice of our personal freedoms does not impose a danger on anyone, limit someone else's freedom, *or prove offensive to those we serve.* As a health care professional, you will be held to high standards in your personal behavior and appearance, so learn to deal with it. I have given you my advice and mean nothing judgmental in what I have written, especially for those not in the medical field. Take it or leave it.

By now, you are thinking, "This fellow is obsessing over cleanliness." Perhaps I am, but with very good reason. Infections can be fearsome to deal with and are still responsible for loss of vision, loss of limbs, and death. Years ago, we operated on a man with a fractured femur and put in an intramedullary rod (a rigid metal rod inserted into the bone marrow canal of the femur) to align the fracture and hold the bone fragments in place for healing. This is not an uncommon procedure and had been done successfully many times in our hospital. The only slightly unusual thing about this patient was that he had suffered from cancer and been treated with chemotherapy in the recent past. The surgery went well, and he was taken back to his room after the normal amount of time in the recovery room. That evening, the surgeon called me to see the patient who had been moved to the intensive care unit and was gravely ill. When I initially saw him, he was febrile and obviously sicker than hell. The leg that had been operated on was completely discolored in a frightening black-and-blue hue. The surgeon told me to lay my hand lightly on his thigh. When I did, I felt the crunching sensation known as crepitus, the telltale sign of gas within the tissues. This clinical picture was compatible with only one diagnosis: gas gangrene. The surgeon was already giving him massive doses of appropriate antibiotics; but despite all our intensive treatment (including removing the intramedullary rod), he died several hours later, the victim of an overwhelming and rapidly progressing infection. We knew that he was undoubtedly immunocompromised because of his history of receiving aggressive chemotherapy, but we were never able to ascertain how the organism responsible for gas gangrene (a *Clostridium* organism) got into this patient. None of us had ever seen an infection come on this quickly and cause death in such a short period of time. It could have been that the organism was in his bowel and that it somehow got into his bloodstream. The surgeon immediately thought that perhaps the intramedullary rod had not been properly sterilized; but all the records, including the tracing of the sterilizer that shows the temperature reached and for how long it is held, confirmed that everything had been done as it should have been. The case remains a tragic mystery, but it illustrates that infections are nothing to joke about and can still occur even with all our best efforts.

In case you still think that I am just obsessing over cleanliness and decorum, let me tell you another true story. I formerly worked with a surgeon, one of the most skilled I ever knew, who had a bit of a God complex—not an unusual finding in physicians in general and surgeons in particular. He was a stinker about sterile technique in the operating room and woe to any nurse who even appeared to break sterility. So far fair dinkum, but this man had a terrible habit of never changing his scrub clothes. He wore them in his office. He wore them home. He usually wore a white coat over them, but not always. As I drove home, I would pass his house, and one day I saw him out cutting the lawn on his riding mower while wearing his OR scrubs. The very next morning, I happened to be in the doctors' locker room when he arrived for surgery. He hung up his white coat and headed for the operating room wearing the same scrubs he had worn the day before and heaven only knows for how many days before that. I stopped him and asked if he had put on fresh scrubs that morning. Looking somewhat sheepish, he replied truthfully and turned around and put on clean scrubs. Fortunately, this man's infection rate was no different than other surgeons. Just the same, there are good reasons for cleanliness in the operating room and everywhere else in the hospital and clinic. Hospitals are already dangerous places because of patients with infections, and we do not need people bringing in more bacteria from pets, lawns, gardens, barns, or wherever. You are right—I am a bit obsessed with cleanliness. I hope you will be too. Wear clean clothes every day!

I made a snide comment in the previous paragraph that I ought to expand on just a bit. This joke will help explain. It seems a fellow passed away and, having lived an exemplary life, arrived in heaven. After being shown to his celestial quarters, he was taken to the cafeteria for supper. While waiting in line along with everyone else, a fellow in a sparkling white lab coat worn over green scrub clothes came rushing into the room and brusquely proceeded to cut in front of everybody, pushing and shoving his way to the head of the line. The new fellow turned to the person next to him and asked, "Gosh, who's that?" The person replied, "Oh, that's just God. He thinks he's a surgeon!"

Generalizations are often inaccurate; nonetheless, surgeons have enjoyed a reputation for pompous behavior since the invention of the scalpel. Sometimes it is deserved, often to the point of being quite comical. A well-known OB/GYN surgeon in Syracuse was so arrogant that he used to say something like this to a new father: "Your wife just gave you a baby boy, son. Thank God for these golden hands!" That was the acme of pomposity in my experience. On the other hand, more than 98 percent of the surgeons I have met in my career are brilliant, skilled, well-humored, kind individuals that I feel privileged to have worked with and proud to call friends. Having told a joke at the expense of the surgeons, I feel compelled to follow up with the surgeon's definition of an anesthesiologist: an anesthesiologist is a doctor who is half-asleep, sitting over a patient who is half-awake. There, we are now even.

One last item about cleanliness: it ought to include your language. There is really no need for foul language in clinics and hospitals, especially when patients are within earshot. You are smart, you are educated, and you would do well to sound like it.

Having said all the above, here is one of my favorite hand-washing stories. Two doctors met in the men's room during a break at a national medical meeting. After enjoying the great relief, one turned and headed for the sink and the other headed for the door. The one going to the sink turned toward the other and said in a tone of condescension, "In Boston, we're taught to wash our hands after we urinate." The one headed for the door turned back with a big grin and replied with a typical Texas drawl: "That's great, Doc! Down there in Dallas, they learn us not to pee on 'em!" I am afraid I have to agree with the Bostonian on this one.

I never yet met a man that I didn't like.
—Will Rogers

Chapter 5

Respect Your Fellow Human Beings

One of the more common responses to "Why do you want to be a doctor?" or "Why do you want to be a nurse?" must be something like this: "So that I can fight disease and help my fellow human beings to have a longer and more pleasant life." Those are marvelous sentiments, of course, but I will wager that the average person who espouses them has yet to meet many of his or her fellow human beings. It is important, therefore, for you to examine your own views of the human race and your place within it.

You do not have to deal directly with human beings in all areas of medicine. In fact, personal contact with patients by physicians varies from the psychiatrist who spends an hour at a time with each patient and develops a strong personal relationship over weeks and months to the pathologist who may never see a complete patient outside of the autopsy room. There are many doctors and nurses in research and administrative roles whose contacts with patients may be quite limited. The same is true in many other allied health fields. For most of us, however, dealing with patients is an everyday experience. You should remember that when you declare yourself a health care professional, you do so to all comers. I have yet to see a shingle or a business card that says, "I treat only the wealthy and the healthy." In all likelihood, you will encounter all kinds of people in your training and after you enter practice. You will see people who are pleasant and nasty, rich and poor, prisoner and police, laborers and managers, old and young, very healthy and very sick, wife beaters and child beaters, saints and sinners, and everyone in between. Notice that I did not mention race, religion, political affiliation, or country of origin. Race is only important insofar as some diseases are more prevalent in specific races. Country of origin is only important in that a patient might be carrying a parasitic or other disease not normally found in the United States. In my opinion, it is one of the lowest forms of human behavior to hate someone for those things that one cannot control: gender, race, or country of origin. It is equally ridiculous to exalt anyone for those attributes alone, qualities over which one has absolutely no control. If people are judged at all, they should be judged solely on their deeds; take heed, however, that it is forbidden to be judgmental in the practice of medicine. Bias, prejudice, and personal hang-ups have no place in treating patients. The only thing we should not tolerate is intolerance. Physicians and all health care professionals cannot practice bigotry. If it bothers you to deal with people who are different from yourself in any way, please find another profession. We are healers, not judges. Our job is to recognize and respect all human beings in need and do all within our power to help those persons.

We must keep our ultimate goal in mind with every patient encountered. That goal is to return each human being to his or her predisease state of functioning. Treating the disease is merely the means of achieving the goal of returning a healthy mother to her family and profession or an electrician to his job site or a minister to his pulpit and so forth. We have to remember that every disease has a person attached. It is the whole person that we must be concerned with, not just a bunch of bacteria, viruses, broken bones, or malignant cells. Unfortunately, it is not always possible, despite our most intense efforts, to achieve the goal of returning the patient to his or her predisease state. This will be a source of frustration for you throughout your career, and it is the source of employment for many trial attorneys, as we shall explore in another chapter.

It is not always easy to take care of patients, and, despite the quote from Will Rogers beginning this chapter, you will not always like or understand those with whom you must deal. This case from my internship days will illustrate the point. I was assigned to emergency room duty. Early one evening, a ten-year-old boy came in with his parents who said that he had fallen off a ladder and hit his head, causing him to lose consciousness for a short while. By the time he arrived at the hospital, he was awake and alert, complaining only of a headache. His neurological examination was within normal limits, and in those days, we had no CT or MRI scan to help us with diagnosing intracranial trauma. Because of the history of loss of consciousness and the height of his fall, I ordered a skull X-ray. It showed that he had a fracture in an extremely delicate area (directly across the path of the middle cerebral artery). We were actually surprised with this finding, because in most instances a simple X-ray of the head is negative in cases like this. I began to suspect that he might have taken a bigger hit than I thought. The combination of the loss of consciousness coupled with the skull fracture in this area dictated that this child be observed in the hospital overnight for monitoring in case delayed intracranial bleeding should occur, something known to happen with fractures in this area. I went to the parents and child, told them the X-ray findings, and explained that we wanted to observe him in the hospital, where urgent care was immediately accessible if required. The father's immediate response was that they were not staying and were taking the child home. I told him quite clearly and truthfully that if they did so, the child might die. He responded angrily, "So what?" I was dumbfounded, having never been confronted with such a cold, heartless attitude to what was clearly a life-or-death situation. In addition, I felt totally helpless because, if the father insisted, there was little I could do to stop him from taking the child away. I approached my supervising resident about getting a court order to allow us to treat the lad appropriately. While we were trying to arrange this, the nurse came and told us that the mother had convinced the father to relent, and he was now agreeing to our admitting the child. Fortunately, the child did well and was discharged the following day with no complications. Because of the father's reaction, we thought of child abuse rather than a fall from a ladder as the cause of this child's skull fracture. In those days, it was not a diagnosis entertained as frequently as it is now, and the liability consequences of a false accusation were significant. Furthermore, there were few social safety nets available in cases of child abuse. Thank goodness, all that has changed. That father's response to my telling him his child might die is something I have never completely gotten over, and it bothers me greatly to this day. Many physicians could tell you other stories like that one and would agree that some patients are easier to treat than others. Most people, however, are wonderful to deal with and thus make the profession so personally rewarding.

The story I have just related reminds me of another case involving strange parental behavior. When I was in the army, I was asked by the pediatricians to help in the care of an infant with pneumonia who was so sick that she required endotracheal intubation and assisted ventilation. The child was critically ill, and we all worked dreadfully hard to keep her alive. After a day or two, the pediatrician suddenly realized that he had not seen the child's parents since the day she was admitted to the hospital. Phone calls to their home went unanswered. Finally, one of the nurses called the father's unit and spoke to his commanding officer. She was told that the soldier was on leave. The parents had dropped the baby off at the hospital and then left on vacation! Fortunately, the child recovered. I do not know what happened to the parents.

How should we deal with our patients? I have always taken the attitude that you should treat other people the way you would like to be treated yourself. That is what the golden rule says, and what could be more simple or authoritative than that? Much of the time, following that rule works and is appreciated by your patients. Some will even ask you, "What would you do, Doc?" Sometimes, however, there is a real clash of ideas between doctor and patient. I will give you a simple theoretical case to help make the point. A patient comes in with a really sore throat and a fever. You do the examination and take a culture that comes back as a streptococcal infection, so-called strep throat. You properly notify the patient and start to write out a prescription for penicillin, still the antibiotic of choice for this disease. The patient stops you and says that he does not want to take an antibiotic. He has read too many articles and heard too much on the news about how doctors overuse antibiotics, and that this is a bad thing (you will learn that yellow journalism does not make your life any easier). So what do you do now? Aspirin or Tylenol will not cure a strep throat. You begin by telling him that this is totally different from treating viral and other nonbacterial conditions with an antibiotic, and that he has a disease for which antibiotic treatment is absolutely the treatment of choice. If that does not work, you tell him all the things that might happen as the result of an untreated strep throat, such as rheumatic fever of the heart, Bright's disease of the kidneys, and even meningitis. If this does not convince him, you may be stuck. In the final analysis, our society dictates that each of us has the right to determine what happens to ourselves, and refusal of medical treatment is one such right. You have to respect the person, even if you do not respect the decision. Too often, we do not really know the wishes of the patient, a problem that surfaces during discussions of end-of-life issues with family members. This is why it is so important for each of us to have a durable power of attorney for health care matters designated, coupled with a so-called living will that spells out our individual wishes for medical treatment in case we are temporarily or permanently unable to make those decisions. Most institutions of medical care now ask patients if they have made such arrangements and request to have copies in their records. They will also help patients to make such arrangements if necessary. If you clearly respect the people who bring themselves to you for care and if they recognize that respect, refusal of treatment is not going to happen very often. Love and respect go hand in hand, and it is paramount that you communicate those feelings to your patients. If you do, you will receive it in kind from them many times over in return.

You will learn that different patients respond in entirely different ways to the same or similar circumstances. You need to remember that and be prepared to manage each as required. I learned this lesson quite clearly the summer before entering medical school when I worked as an orderly at St. Mary's Hospital in Rochester before Arline and I got married. I was technically a float and was assigned to a different floor each day. I especially liked the surgical floors, but my favorite assignment was the emergency room. One day, two little girls about ten years old came in at the same time. One was screaming and fussing and being totally obnoxious, while the other was quiet and sat motionless with her arms carefully folded in front of her. The screamer had a tiny little laceration that she got from falling on a stick. It was gaping a bit, and today would have been repaired with Steri-Strips. But we did not have them in those days, so she needed a stitch. In order to accomplish this, we had to restrain the child on what is called a papoose board; and while that dealt with her kicking and fighting, it did nothing to lessen her screams. After she had been successfully treated and began to quiet down, I went to the other girl who still had not let out a peep.

I looked at her and asked, "What's wrong with you, honey?"

She looked at me and replied with a big sigh in a resigned, matter-of-fact manner, "Oh, I broke my clavicle again!"

The X-ray proved her right. I could not imagine the degree of difference in pain between a tiny laceration and a broken bone, especially the clavicle, yet the reactions of these children were 180 degrees from what I would have expected. You will also learn that the behavior of children quite often, but not uniformly, will mirror the reactions of the adults who accompany them, as was true in these cases. If Mom and Dad have it together, the child quite often will have it together also. If Mom and Dad are going berserk, expect the child to act the same. It would be a dull existence if we were all the same. We are not.

Sometimes patients require and benefit from service beyond what they will teach you in school. My longtime friend and Episcopal priest, Paul Goodland, used to refer to special, unexpected, and random deeds of kindness as "acts of supererogation." Such acts are often necessary in medicine, and sometimes they can be amazingly therapeutic. Early in my practice, I helped take care of an older nurse who worked at a small hospital several miles from ours. She normally worked the 3:00 p.m. to 11:00 p.m. shift at her hospital, and one night she fell asleep coming home from work and drove into a bridge abutment. In addition to fracturing both of her legs, she also fractured her jaw. In critical condition and needing specialized care, she was quickly transferred to our facility, where she spent several hours in the operating room for both orthopedic and dental surgery. When it was over, she was taken to the intensive care unit in traction and with her jaws wired shut. She remained in intensive care for several days during which I saw her in consultation for continuing care. After she was transferred to a regular room, I continued to drop in on her to monitor her progress and to say hello. The nurses told me that she had not had many visitors other than her son. She was destined to be in the hospital for many weeks due to her injuries, because she needed to be in traction until such time as it was appropriate to put her in a spica cast, one that includes both legs and the pelvis. Because her jaw was wired shut, her diet consisted of liquid that was both monotonous and bland.

You have probably not been in traction, and it is equally unlikely that you have had your jaw wired shut. These are not pleasant predicaments. The human brain has an inordinate amount of volume devoted to the tongue. It is an important organ, one that we use incessantly, freely, and most often unthinkingly. Envision your jaws being wired shut and your tongue being caged behind your teeth. Imagine further your inability to take in solid food, chew it, and enjoy its taste. Limiting the function of the human tongue is a bit like tying one's hands behind one's back. Now picture your lower body being trapped in devices that put weight on your legs to pull fractured bone fragments into alignment and hold them there until healing occurs. Remember that the desired therapeutic effect can only be achieved with your body in one position—on your back. How well can you sleep on your back all night long? How would it be to lie on your back all day and all night without any possibility of turning to the side or onto your tummy, even for a moment? Finally, imagine being in this predicament not for a day or a week but for months. Sound like torture? It certainly is, even though its intent is completely humane and therapeutic. Few patients experience this condition without developing some degree of depression, and this patient was no exception.

One day when I stopped in to see her, she was crying. The whole situation was finally getting to her. She told me that she would feel a lot better if only she could get something to eat that had some flavor. As the father of three small children, I immediately thought of some of the foods we gave them as infants. Baby food in general is not especially flavorful, but some of it is delicious. I remember especially enjoying little tastes of a couple of the fruity desserts, one being like Dutch apple pie and the other being something called Blueberry Buckle. I asked my wife if she could pick up a couple of jars of each when she did her shopping, and then I took them to the patient. She was able to squeeze the baby food through her wired jaws, and she loved them; moreover, for a while, her spirits really picked up. I made sure to keep her supplied.

Eventually, she began to become depressed again. This time, I had seen a poster in another patient's room. It depicted a little man sitting on a toilet, and the caption read, "I'm so happy here, I could just shit!" With that patient's permission, I made a copy of it and took it to her. I taped it to the wall and, as I backed away, she read it and burst into laughter. She kept it hanging there, but again became depressed some time later. As fate would have it, I saw another poster in a different patient's room. This one had two buzzards sitting on a bare tree branch looking horrifically menacing. The caption read, "Patience, my ass! I'm going to kill somebody." Now I knew the patient who owned this poster very well. He was a crusty old fellow with an equally crusty sense of humor. He delighted in my making a copy of the picture for someone else. When I hung it in her room, I thought that she would laugh herself out of traction.

Ultimately, she did well and was discharged from the hospital. I am pretty certain that she returned to work. Please do not think that humor is the most important treatment for depression, because severe depression is a very serious disease. Situational depression such as she was experiencing can respond to humor and other kinds of diversions, and that is exactly what she needed. This is the sort of situation where the nurse's care becomes at least as important as the doctor's. Kindness, understanding, sympathy, humor, big smiles, and lots of tender loving care are all required to nurse these patients back to health. Two lessons can be taken from this experience: (1) acts of supererogation are inexpensive and greatly appreciated, and (2) there are effective treatments other than pills and injections.

You should respect your colleagues. Medicine is a difficult pursuit, and we need to support each other. If someone is doing a good job, it is always appropriate to say so. A verbal pat on the back is greatly appreciated in my experience, and it is not offered as often as it should be. We ought to be there for each other to help whenever it is needed in whatever way is appropriate. Hallway consultations and lunchtime "grand rounds" are part of the camaraderie of being part of a team and often benefit patients immensely. Always try to be quick to help and slow to criticize. Be careful of passing judgment on your colleagues. We are all capable of making mistakes, and most of us do so from time to time. There is a difference, however, between the honest, infrequent mistake and a pattern of ineptitude or willful misbehavior. Earlier, I said that we should be supportive of each other, but that does not mean that we should ignore unacceptable behavior or practice. There are well-defined avenues for reporting and investigating grievances. It is far more preferable to use these avenues than to apply personal confrontation. I have had experience using both, and you can take it from me that the former is preferable to the latter. Fortunately, despite what you read in the headlines or see on TV, true malpractitioners are relatively rare. In my years of practice, I have observed that the great majority of physicians and other health care providers are wonderful people to be around because they are competent, hardworking, honest individuals dedicated to the well being of their patients.

We need to respect all our fellow health care practitioners, including physician assistants, nurses, nurse anesthetists, paramedics, pharmacists, radiology technicians, lab technicians, OR technicians, orderlies, receptionists, and all others who help us take care of patients. None of us can function totally alone. Practicing medicine requires a lot of specialized help. I have been impressed by the skill and dedication of those who help me, and I have the utmost admiration for them. Medical students climb the "magic ladder" of increasing status from lowly med student to slightly higher resident to slightly higher chief resident to attending physician. The "magic ladder" is nothing but age-old foolishness in my view, yet it is the source of one of my favorite jokes. It seems that the cardiology team was making hospital rounds and had just seen a patient who had suffered a heart attack. As they were discussing the case in the hallway, the question arose as to when patients should be advised to resume sexual relations after having had a major heart attack. The chief of cardiology in his typical pontificating manner said that it should be a jolly long time, because intercourse is 100 percent work. The junior attending physician disagreed, stating that intercourse is only 75 percent work and 25 percent pleasure. The chief resident piped in saying that in his opinion it is 50 percent work and 50 percent pleasure. At this, the first-year resident, feeling somewhat uncomfortable in disagreeing with his superiors, opined that it is 25 percent work and 75 percent pleasure. Finally, the lowly intern, looking thoroughly disgusted with the whole conversation, loudly proclaimed, "Gentlemen, we all know that intercourse is 100 percent pleasure, because if there were *any* work involved, you all would have me doing it for you!"

Forgive me, but that joke reminds me of something that really happened at Strong Memorial Hospital. The chief of cardiology was a man named Paul Yu, who was of Chinese descent. He was a wonderful man and superb physician. He was known around the world and was the editor of one of the important journals in his specialty. It was the custom at Strong for the cardiology and cardiac surgery teams to make weekly combined rounds to see patients recovering from open-heart surgery. The two teams totaled a dozen or more people. Several of the cardiology fellows studying under Dr. Yu happened to be oriental that year. As they approached the bed of a gentleman who had undergone aortic valve replacement surgery a few days earlier, one of the surgical residents shook his shoulder and asked, "Mr. Jones! Do you know where you are this morning?"

The man, who had been mildly disoriented since surgery, slowly opened his eyes and looked toward the foot of his bed where he saw Dr. Yu and several other people with Asian faces. He looked back to the surgical resident and said, "Oh, I don't know—Tokyo?" As all the participants were now convulsing with uncontrollable laughter, the rounds were suspended.

I have never cared much for hierarchy. We are all diligently scrambling for the benefit of the patient, and we should treat each other equally and with respect. A physician should never look upon a nurse as someone stupid and vice versa. In fact, many nurses are a lot smarter than many doctors and a heck of a lot more experienced. If they are so smart, why don't they go to medical school, a doctor might ask? Because they want to be nurses and are essential and important doing what they do, that's why. This is not a slave state, yet. If they wanted to go to medical school, they would. Be thankful that they do not, because quite often the sick human being is more dependent on the nurse than on the doctor, as I have already pointed out. Remember also that the hospital and clinic staffs are examples of teamwork. There are no superstars, although you are likely to find several who think they are. Each member of the team is as important as the next. That is why I have always greeted the janitor with as much enthusiasm and warmth as the hospital administrator. I challenge you to try working without either. Can you imagine what a hospital would look like without proper janitorial services? Furthermore, I will wager that finding a replacement for a good janitor is harder than finding a good administrator. I have been fortunate where I have worked because in addition to feeling like I am a member of a team, I have also felt like I am a member of a family. Get to know your coworkers and their families, respect them, help them, and reward them. You will be surprised how nice life can be and how much can get done when everyone pulls in the same direction. Before condemning anyone, consider the old saying about walking a mile in someone else's shoes. Could you do as well as the person you are criticizing under similar circumstances?

For you future and current physicians, do not let your head get too big because you have gone to medical school. We treat the sick and sometimes work unspeakably hard, but there are others out there who work just as hard, get paid less, and make our society as wonderful as it is with their endeavors. Think of the service men and women, police, and firefighters who daily put their lives in danger for all of us. Be grateful for the truckers who deliver all our goods at the expense of huge amounts of time away from home and family. When you are cooped up in a hospital or clinic all day long, it is easy to forget that there is a whole world of people out there doing their various things to keep our civilization moving along, and that they are just as important in the great scheme of life as you are. A good many of them have knowledge and skills of which I am quite envious. I watch the version of *A Christmas Carol* starring George C. Scott as Ebenezer Scrooge every year. The messages that come through most loudly to me are that in the sight of God, everyone is important, and that money is only important for providing necessities, for the enjoyment of life, and for doing as much good as possible. If you get to feeling really superior because of what you do, remember that the workers in the city's sewer and water treatment systems save more lives by their toil in a week than you will in your entire lifetime. Contemplate for a moment that the money invested in a single renal dialysis unit would provide numerous water and sewage projects in developing nations and save thousands of lives of all ages each year. Respect your fellow human beings, and give thanks that you are a member of this incredible species. Contribute all that you can and be grateful for all that you receive.

If you just communicate you can get by.
But if you skillfully communicate, you can work miracles.
—Jim Rohn

Words are, of course, the most powerful drug used by mankind.
—Rudyard Kipling

Chapter 6

Communication

A major asset of our species is the ability to communicate with each other in great detail, a gift as important as intelligence itself. There are so many different ways to share ideas and emotions that we sometimes forget that art, music, and mathematics are just as important as words. Without communication, our collective intelligence would be greatly diminished and we ourselves would suffer, because the need to express ourselves seems as fundamental as our needs to eat, drink, and breathe. We humans can harvest the fruits of our cerebral hemispheres and deliver them to other individuals, allowing us to escape our shells and reach out to the world in ways unique to our species. This capability is as important a distinguishing characteristic of our kind as the opposable thumb and upright posture. The explosion in communication technology during my lifetime is one of the biggest miracles I have seen, ranking up there with our ability to journey away from the home planet, a journey that would be essentially useless without our capacity to learn and tell others about it. We do not always use our abilities in this area appropriately, which is unfortunate because mistakes in sharing information can be deadly. Precise communication in medicine, as in other professions, is essential for our being able to complete our goals successfully.

One evening, as a resident, I was making rounds to see patients having surgery the following day. As I entered a nursing station, I saw a nurse with a collection of 1 mL ampoules lined up on the counter, and one by one, she was breaking them open and drawing them up in a large syringe.

I walked over and, out of curiosity, looked at one of the ampoules. It said Levophed, which is the trade name of norepinephrine, a neurotransmitter and hormone secreted by the sympathetic nervous system. Its effects are to raise the blood pressure by narrowing small arteries in the body as well as to stimulate the heart. When used in emergency medicine, which it rarely is these days, it is administered by diluting 1 mg (the contents of 1 mL) in 500 mL of saline solution and giving it by slow intravenous infusion with careful monitoring of the heart rate and blood pressure. The dose must be carefully titrated to achieve the desired effects. This is an extremely potent medication with dramatic results, and it is quite dangerous if improperly given; in fact, one of its nicknames is Lethophed, implying the potential lethality of this substance. I asked the nurse what she was doing. She replied that a doctor had ordered her patient to receive 15 mg of Levophed by intramuscular injection, so she was drawing up the requisite 15 mL to give the woman. I had never heard of giving Levophed in such a large amount or by intramuscular injection and knew this was irrational and prohibitively dangerous. I asked to see the order that the doctor had written. I looked at the order sheet in the patient's chart, and there was an order for a drug called Levoprome, not Levophed. Levoprome is a nonnarcotic analgesic, a sedative, and an antipsychotic. This doctor's handwriting was not the best, but it was legible enough that Levoprome did not look much like Levophed. The dosage ordered was perfectly appropriate for Levoprome. It is probable that this nurse had seen L-e-v-o-p . . . and immediately read it as Levophed. Misreading is something that we are all capable of doing, which is why it is so important to recheck to be certain that we are doing the right thing. What troubled me is that she did not question the order nor verify it with a colleague. Levophed is never given in the quantity or the route ordered for Levoprome. This should have raised the proverbial red flag in her mind to the point of making her contact the doctor for a clarification. Had I not come along at that moment, she might have given that patient a huge dose of the wrong medicine with predictably fatal results. I showed the nurse the order, explained the difference between the two drugs, and described the possible consequences of her giving the patient so much Levophed. I watched her discard what she had drawn up. By the way, the manner in which medications are handled in hospitals now makes this sort of thing much less likely to occur.

Why would a nurse not call a doctor to clarify an order? He or she might be clueless, but that will be pretty rare because the greatest number of nurses I have known are astute and compulsively careful. Fatigue leads to mistakes, a problem that plagues us all. A nurse may be distracted and overly busy, something that happens more often than it should in large institutions with many patients and inadequate staffing. The worst reason is that the nurse may be afraid to call the doctor. That may sound crazy, but I have seen it more than once. Many times, I have been at a nursing station and have been asked if I could read a doctor's order. If I clearly can, I do; but if not, I tell the nurse to call the doctor. So many times, I have heard the reply, "Oh, he doesn't like to be bothered, and he'll yell." My response has always been along the lines of "Tough, call him anyway! If he yells, it's his problem, not yours." Doctors who write illegibly deserve to be called night and day for clarification of orders. Perhaps they will take the time to write better if they are bugged enough. I knew one physician who refused to take a call from any nurse other than the house supervisor, the nurse with overall supervision of the whole nursing staff of the hospital. That attitude is not only arrogant and idiotic, but is also utterly dangerous.

Failure to communicate because of fear is dangerous. A surgeon I once knew could be frighteningly bombastic, which caused many of the nursing staff to feel petrified of him, even though he was a pussycat at heart. He was knowledgeable, gifted as a surgeon, and quite lovable in his way; nonetheless, he could scare the dickens out of nurses and anyone else who let him get away with it.

Let me interrupt myself yet again to advise you never to be afraid of someone with a big, loud mouth. Feel free to fear someone wielding a .357 magnum and waving it under your nose, but someone who shouts a lot is simply a noisemaker, so do not let that person scare you. Now if he or she happens to be the boss, the chairman of your department, or some other big shot, you may fear for your position because of this person's obnoxious trait; however, it is better to be fired for wanting to do the right thing than to keep your job and do the wrong thing because of someone who likes to bellow or because of fear of being fired.

OK, back to my story. This surgeon operated on a patient's sinuses. It was a fairly difficult and bloody procedure, so she was admitted for observation. In the recovery room, this patient's left eye began to swell a bit and become discolored. No one notified the surgeon or the anesthesiologist, something I have never understood because none of us in the anesthesia department were at all frightening to anyone and our recovery room nurses were superb. The patient was taken to her room, a report was given, and swelling and discoloration of the eye, now much more apparent, was duly noted in the nurse's notes. Again, no one called the surgeon. By suppertime, the patient complained that she could not see out of her eye, which by this time was swollen shut and quite discolored with the typical appearance of a major shiner, but still no one bothered to report this important development to the surgeon. In the morning, the surgeon came into her room to check on her progress. Imagine his horror at seeing a severely swollen eye that looked as if she had taken a punch from Muhammad Ali. In addition, when with considerable effort, he retracted the lids to look at the eyeball, the pupil was dilated and unreactive; and the patient could not see out of it at all. We took the patient to the operating room right away to decompress her orbit (eye socket), which had filled with blood, but her vision was irretrievably lost due to the pressure in her orbit shutting off the blood supply to the optic nerve and retina. If the nurses had alerted the surgeon to the situation early when swelling was initially noted, the patient's vision in that eye might have been saved. Unfortunately, the nurses all down the line were loath to call him because their previous experiences with him on the phone had been so unpleasant. The patient did not sue the doctor. She did sue the hospital, because the nurses did not listen to her when she told them that she could not see out of her eye.

Why had the patient been admitted to the hospital in the first place? It was for monitoring for possible bleeding. The nurses saw the swelling around the eye and noticed the blue discoloration of her eyelids, but they did not notify the surgeon. This was a classic breakdown in communications, for which both the nurses and the surgeon were at fault. I beg you fledgling physicians to treat nurses and all others who "bother" you at inconvenient times with kindness and respect. If you must correct someone, please do it in person and in a rational and adult manner, not screaming like a maniac. Screaming is a form of communication; but in the long run, it is counterproductive, potentially harmful, and most often childish. Used sparingly and appropriately, it can be effective, but those instances ought to be rare. To you fledgling nurses, I would advise that you never be afraid to call the doctor no matter how obnoxious his or her reputation.

I must confess to acting out childishly over the phone on one occasion at the end of my first year of practice in Iowa. I had been on call by myself for a whole month while my senior partner was on vacation and before our new third partner had started. It had been a busy month, and I was bushed. On a Sunday afternoon, the phone rang and the nursing supervisor asked if I could come to the hospital to start an intravenous on a patient of one of my internist partners. She made the mistake of telling me that she did not ask the internist himself to do it because he had been on call all weekend, and she thought he might be tired. I blew my stack. Boy, I was hot. The nerve of this person, who knew quite well that I had been on call for a month, really annoyed me, and I unloaded both barrels. The intravenous was not for an emergency, so I told her I would take care of it later in the afternoon when I came to the hospital for my evening rounds. Later, the nursing supervisor of the three-to-eleven shift called me and said that she had started the intravenous, and that I need not worry about it. She also apologized for her colleague's lack of tact earlier in the day. Evidently, she had received a full report of my ranting and raving on the phone. I, in turn, apologized for acting out, but she assured me that her colleague had asked for it. That was the only time I ever blew my stack over the phone, except at telemarketers.

Today, written communication is improving by use of the electronic medical record. Mistakes will still be made if we are not extremely careful, but errors due to lousy penmanship should at least be reduced. Computers and electronic medical records are great, but not everyone has them yet; furthermore, we will be writing by hand in the record into the foreseeable future, perhaps until such time that we can reliably dictate to the computers that write our electronic records. I have to tell you that my handwriting is quite legible, even at my advanced age and even though I am left-handed. I blush to brag that I won a certificate for excellent penmanship in the sixth grade at Springdale Elementary School in Tulsa, Oklahoma. My writing is not as good as it was then, but you can still read it easily. I have had to read others' dreadful handwriting since I started medical school, and you can take it to the bank that perusing a handwritten medical record can be a real chore. I remember in medical school picking up the chart of a neurosurgical patient and starting to read the neurosurgeon's note. Initially, I was delighted that the writing was so incredibly elegant and neat. All the letters were of uniform size and precisely spaced. Here surely was a note I could handle. Quickly, my delight turned to horror; the handwriting was completely illegible. It might as well have been written in Chinese. I said something to one of the nurses, who told me that his writing was always the same and that no one could read it. I was appalled. Years later, I knew a general practitioner who worked for our clinic and saw patients coming in without appointments for a variety of problems. He was a delightful man, kind and knowledgeable, and perfectly fit for the difficult job he was asked to do. I never heard an unkind word about him, except for his handwriting. It was atrocious. Everybody knew it, including him, but he could not improve it, even though he tried. One day, he was found going up and down the halls of the clinic with a chart in his hand, asking nurses and other doctors if they could read his note! The next day, the clinic administrator bought him a typewriter and from then on he typed everything, which delighted everyone who had to read his notes, especially him. Written communication is important, whether it be writing prescriptions, notes in the chart, or nursing orders in the hospital. Use the computer when you can, but otherwise make certain that your handwriting is legible.

It is hard to overemphasize the importance and utility of the medical record, an instrument of communication that is becoming even better with the advent of computer-based systems. As an anesthesiologist, I like to know as much about my patients as I can before meeting them face-to-face. I have pored through thousands and thousands of patients' records over the years reading barely legible handwriting and puzzling over abbreviations known only to the author; nonetheless, I have gained a tremendous amount of knowledge in doing so, much of it to the benefit of the patients for whom I would be giving care. The quality of information in the record varies from superb to unconscionable. I have seen consultation notes that would make excellent contributions to a textbook, complete with references to the current literature. I have seen charts in which the patient's physician has not written a single syllable after several days of hospitalization. Most records lie somewhere between these two extremes. Here are a few recommendations based on my years of reading records, and these recommendations are germane for anyone making a note in a medical record:

1. Make your entries meaningful, concise, accurate, and complete.
2. Make your entries legible to all, not just to yourself.
3. Record the time and date of your entry and make a note each time you see the patient for other than pure social reasons.
4. If you record that you are going to do something (i.e., order a test), be sure that you do it and that you follow up on it.

5. Make certain that you are recording in the proper chart. It is easier to make mistakes than you can imagine.
6. Do not initiate battles in the chart between yourself and others caring for the same patient. I have seen such disagreements heatedly recorded in charts, and it is not pretty. It is also incredibly stupid, because medical-legally, it is like shooting yourself in the foot at best and like signing a blank check at worst. This practice is entirely unprofessional, unscientific, and unjustified, so do not do it. If you have a beef with your colleague, pick up the phone or walk down the hall and talk. You will find that to be a much more productive and professional way of handling disagreements.
7. Keep your charting up to date. Getting behind in the paperwork is a terrible habit to get into, a dreadful habit to break, and a good way to lose your hospital privileges. Like it or not, paperwork is necessary, expected of you, and taken very seriously by those in a position to hurt you professionally and financially. I have seen too many physicians get into big trouble because they did not do their paperwork in a timely fashion. It is not an easy task, but a necessary one. Electronic medical records should facilitate the process.
8. Make certain that whatever you note in the record is truthful. Falsification of medical records is a serious offense. Honesty, even if it hurts, is far superior to fabrication.
9. When you have written something in the record, reread it and imagine someone reading it back to you at a peer review committee meeting or, better yet, in a court of law. This will help you remember to avoid using pejorative language you might later regret.
10. Sign your name legibly. Take a lesson from John Hancock.

One of the delightful aspects of communication is "shop talk." We all like to talk about our triumphs and tragedies (if we're honest); and in doing so, we learn a lot from each other. Medical education is an ongoing challenge for us all, and casual conversations can be an important part of the process. When the conversation involves talking about a patient, we need to be exceedingly careful. Hallway consultations can be quite helpful, but they should be done in a way to hide a patient's identity and to ensure that no one is listening, especially family members. This is also true of comments made at the table in the cafeteria at lunch or dinner. You never know who is sitting at the next table, and it might be a family member of the patient you are discussing. Privacy of information is very important, something you will hear much about in your training and practice. I will tell you a brief story from my own experience to illustrate. As a medical student, I was about to do a history and physical on an elderly gentleman scheduled for prostate surgery on the following day. His room was filled with family members, so I asked them to wait in the hall while I did my examination. I politely shut the door after they had all stepped outside. As I took his history, it was clear that he was extremely hard of hearing. As part of a good urologic workup, I had to ask him questions about sexually transmitted diseases.

I said to him, "Have you ever had syphilis?"

He replied by cupping his hand behind his ear and saying, "Huh?"

Then I said a little louder, "Have you ever had gonorrhea?"

Again he replied, "Huh?"

This time, much louder so that he could definitely hear me, I asked, "Have you ever had the clap?"

With a look of panic on his face, he suddenly put his outstretched index finger in front of his pursed lips and said, "Shhhhhhhhh!" Then, pointing to the door, he added, "They don't know!" Be careful what you say, where you say it, and to whom you say it.

We make a big issue out of identifying the correct operative side these days. This is an essential thing to do, because nobody wants to cut off the wrong leg or operate on a perfectly healthy eye. The current custom is to have the surgeon mark the operative side on the day of surgery. At the time of surgery, a "time out" is taken, which means that everyone stops to identify the patient once again and to confirm which side is being operated on and which procedure is being performed. If people do this as compulsively as they should, wrong side and wrong procedure accidents ought to disappear. Many years ago, a patient was scheduled for a lumbar laminectomy to remove a ruptured disc. I noted that the patient, who was anesthetized by one of the nurse anesthetists at our institution, had been put to sleep and placed facedown on the special rack used for that procedure and all seemed to be going as planned. Shortly afterward, I checked into the room and saw that the patient had been taken off the rack, placed on his back, and that the endotracheal tube previously placed in his windpipe had been removed. The patient was waking up and moaning. I asked the anesthetist if anything had gone wrong. He replied that when the surgeon came into the room, he noted that the patient's leg had not been marked by the nursing supervisor the night before, so he ordered the anesthetist to wake the patient up so he could find out which side he was supposed to operate on. I was furious beyond words and confronted the surgeon in no uncertain terms that he should not have done that. I reminded him clearly that it was his responsibility to know which side to operate on, not the night supervisor's. It was folly to ask a patient just awakening from anesthesia which side is supposed to be operated on. That is like asking a stone-cold drunk the value of pi to six significant figures. Even if he gives you some numbers, how are you going to believe him? Here was an example of a breakdown of communications with the potential for extremely serious consequences. In the introduction of this book, I referred to bad apples spoiling the barrel. This surgeon was the single most rotten apple I ever worked with, and you will read more about him if you read on. Happily, this patient did well. The surgeon's communication skills remained lousy. I have interviewed scores of his patients and asked what surgery they were going to have. Many replied, "I don't know. Doc just said I needed to have an operation, that's all, so here I am." I have never been able to figure out how an otherwise sane and intelligent patient could be so naïve as to accept surgery with such limited information. He was the only surgeon I have ever dealt with who was truculent in so many areas.

I have saved the most important issue about communication for last: communicate with your patients. There are many facets to the doctor-patient relationship, but none is more important than clear, thorough communication in both directions. This goes for others too, especially nurses and paramedics. In order to make a proper diagnosis, you must have a thorough history of the present and past illnesses, and you must learn how to get that history from the patient or family member. Most often, it requires asking multiple questions, but it also requires good listening skills. When the history has been taken and the physical examination completed, you will have a list of possible diagnoses in your mind that will guide you to further investigations. Let's look at a couple of ways in which this can be related to the patient:

"Mr. Babcock, I think you might have a carcinoma causing your symptoms. So we're going to do some tests, including an MRI, metabolic screen, CBC, and chest film, just to see if this thing has already metastasized."

Is there anything wrong with this? The doctor sounds smart enough but has made some common and serious mistakes. First of all, he has used medical terms that may be totally foreign to the patient. Do not assume that the average patient recognizes the term "carcinoma," as you certainly will by the time you finish your training. Many patients will recognize the term "MRI" (magnetic resonance imaging) but may have only a vague notion of what it is or what it does. Metabolic screen is simply a series of tests done on a sample of blood that gives us information about liver and kidney functions, among others, but the phrase itself may be meaningless to a patient. A CBC is a complete blood count and gives a lot of information about the effects blood loss might have had as well as about the function of the bone marrow. Abbreviations like CBC are quite useful to us in medicine, but they are totally inappropriate to use when talking to a patient. Physicians use the jargon "chest film" frequently to refer to a chest X-ray, but the patient may have no idea what it means. It may sound to the patient like he's going to have a picture taken of his chest. "And would that be with my shirt on or off, Doc?" Finally, few will recognize the term "metastasized" unless they are associated with the medical field or have had someone in the family with cancer.

There are other problems besides using too much medical jargon. Using the term "we're going to" is less desirable than "we'd like to." It is the patient's body, after all, and the patient ought to be brought into the decision-making process. There is nothing to be lost and everything to be gained in doing so. The doctor has also been a bit blunt and even premature in using the terms "carcinoma" and "metastasized," even though they may fit into his differential diagnosis. Patients need time to assimilate information, especially when it is thrown at them in as confusing a way as this has been. Even if we suspect the worst, it is our responsibility to maintain a level of optimism and hope that will sustain the patient in the potentially tough times ahead. Here is another way to communicate this:

"Mr. Babcock, I'm a little worried about your symptoms, because serious tumors can sometimes cause this sort of thing. I'd like to do some further testing, including an MRI, which is a special test done in the X-ray department that will give us a pretty clear picture of what's going on inside of you. I think it would also be wise to do some blood tests just to ensure that your major organs like the liver and kidneys are functioning properly and also do a complete blood count to see if you are anemic as a result of the bleeding you described to me. I also think you need to have an X-ray of your chest in view of your smoking history and your exposure to asbestos many years ago. If you agree, we can set up the appointments to do all these things at your convenience. Perhaps you have some questions about all this that I could try to answer for you."

This time, the medical jargon is minimal, and there is a hint of compassion that was missing in the first example. There are also simple explanations of why the doctor wants to do the tests, and by saying "I'd like to," he is asking the patient's permission to proceed. There are more words in this example compared with the first, but the small amount of time needed to be more thorough and compassionate is of little consequence compared with the good it will do in the long run. We should always give the patient an opportunity to ask questions. All of us in medicine ought to be good teachers, and our most important students are our patients. Suppose the patient says, "Do you think that I have cancer, Doc?" The doctor in the first example might reply, "Yes, that's what I'm afraid of." The doctor in the second example might say, "That certainly is a possibility, but it is really too early to know. Let's do these tests and find out what they can tell us. After that, we'll talk, because then we'll have a little better idea of what we're dealing with. Fair enough?" The first doctor has just scared the crap out of his patient. The second has held out hope and offered further justification for the tests he wants to perform.

I know this all sounds simple enough, but when you are in training, you work so hard to learn the language of medicine that by the time you graduate, you think everybody knows those fancy words also. They don't. Do not forget plain English while you are learning the language you will need to know to be a health care provider. At the same time, never talk down to the patient. Remember to whom you are talking when seeing a patient, and do your best to present things in a manner that this person can understand. It is important if you suspect something really bad is going on to be especially compassionate in the way you present your suspicions to the patient, and always offer as much hope as you can. If you do, you will be very popular, effective, and successful.

It would be difficult to overemphasize the importance of good communication between you and the patient. I hope that you have entered medical training to learn to serve the suffering. The first thing I want you to learn is, Talk to Your Patients! The second thing to learn is, Listen to Your Patients! The third thing is, Be Compassionate! Please do not become an automaton stuffed with medical knowledge and skills but unable to relate in any warm, humanly way to those you serve. I have observed several practitioners guilty of being robot like in my years of practice and, if given a choice, I would not choose to have them treat my family or me. You are a human being dealing with human beings, often at the most difficult times in life. Learn to lean on your humanity and to treat your patients accordingly.

There is another aspect of patient communication that is totally different from when I started practice, a time when there were no personal computers and no Internet. Now any person with a connection to the World Wide Web has virtually infinite access to information, both good and bad, using only a search engine and a few keystrokes. This will have important consequences for you and your patients. It is possible that your patients may be extremely well informed before they come to you. It is also possible that they may be tragically ill informed. You, of course, will have to stay knowledgeable and current to distinguish between the two.

I need to say a bit more about listening to the patient. We are often presented with situations or symptoms that are confusing to say the least. I will give you a couple of examples to illustrate. We once had a man in the recovery room who had undergone repair of a hernia and hydrocoele (a collection of fluid around the testis). When he awoke from the anesthetic, he began to moan loudly. Despite being given what should have been adequate amounts of painkillers, he continued to make the same loud noise of discomfort and would not answer us when asked directly what was bothering him nor say anything else even though he appeared wide awake. We were about to write this man off as an oddball when the surgeon happened by and decided to look at the man's wound. The dressing was being held on with a scrotal support, and as soon as the support was released, the man stopped making noise and gave a great sigh of relief. The scrotal support had simply been applied too tightly! I have yet to figure out why he couldn't have just told us that.

In another incident, a woman who had undergone laparoscopic pelvic surgery was unusually uncomfortable in the recovery room, and her symptoms were atypical. She went from having lower abdominal cramps (not uncommon) to having severe back pain associated with nausea and vomiting. She too had received substantial doses of an opioid painkiller without appreciable relief. She complained that the pain felt just as it had when she had been in labor. When the nurse called the surgeon to tell him about the patient's back pain, his only response was, "I didn't operate on her back!" He had written her off as a nut. This was unfortunate, because a little while later, her anesthesiologist gave her a different kind of painkiller, a nonsteroidal anti-inflammatory drug, and her symptoms immediately cleared. Her symptoms had probably been due to marked uterine cramping, and the second painkiller had undoubtedly acted to relax the uterus, one of its known effects.

The point of those two stories is that you have to listen carefully to the patient and do all that you can to sort out the complaints. Life does not always come in the neat little packages described in textbooks or in professors' lectures. Sometimes multiple entities occur at the same time, blurring lines and resulting in confusing signs. When you have listened to all the symptoms, examined all the physical findings, perused all the laboratory results, and still do not have an answer, ask a colleague for help. Two heads are often better than one, and many times, it requires more than two. When the clinical picture is not clear, please do not excuse your inability to make the diagnosis by declaring that the patient is a whacko. That should be the last possible diagnosis entertained and only after the exclusion of all the others. The corollary, of course, is that whackos get sick too, so you still have to listen to them.

It has been said that the sweetest sound to the human ear is the sound of one's own name. The author of such a statement must never have heard an aria or a symphony; nonetheless, it is a well-made point that our names are precious to us. It is a common practice these days for clerks and others to address people by their first names. I remember that a student once asked my wife her first name. Her response was, "Mrs.!" Our generation continues to feel that it is disrespectful for a young person to call an older person by his or her first name. This is especially true in a medical setting where you are often already stripped of your dignity by taking off your clothes and being forced into a skimpy, ill-fitting examination gown, following which some friendly young person comes in and calls you by your first name, adding to your nakedness. Please give all patients the respect they deserve by addressing them with their title and last name. If they subsequently ask you to call them by their first name, it is acceptable to do so, especially when a long-term relationship has been established. I am also offended when a bank teller asks, "So, Gary, what are you going to do today?" It is none of his damn business what I am going to do, and he does not know me well enough to call me Gary. I probably sound like a miserable old sourpuss, but I am not. It is simply that there is something called etiquette, and many in the current generation have forgotten that it exists. I encourage you to be polite and to treat people with dignity and good manners.

Do not forget to communicate with the patient's family. Unless there is a communication problem of any kind, it is most often wise to examine a patient alone or in the presence of a nurse or physician's assistant; but it is better to speak with the patient in the presence of the spouse, parent, child, or other family member when you are ready to discuss the diagnostic and treatment options. For simple things, this is not always necessary, but for major illnesses, it certainly is. In this day of outpatient surgery, it is mandatory to have a significant other present when giving postoperative instructions, because the patient may remember amazingly little of that conversation due to the effects of sedatives and anesthetics. Those instructions must also be given in writing, a good idea for instructions given in the doctor's office as well. The nurses I have been fortunate enough to work with have been excellent when giving postoperative instructions, and the patients really appreciate it. Remembering the family is a good idea not only for compassionate but also for practical reasons, because involving the spouse or other caregiver in the therapeutic process often means that things will be done properly, such as filling prescriptions and taking medications as directed. In addition, each patient is deserving of an advocate, someone dedicated to his or her best interests. A spouse or child may well be inclined to ask important questions that the patient either does not think of or is reluctant to ask. Naturally, it is expected that you will get the patient's permission before sharing information with anyone, even a spouse. It is decidedly unusual to be denied that permission, but not unknown.

I will end my thoughts on communication by advising you to use common sense at all times. Keep in mind how incredibly important proper communication is and act accordingly. How would you like to be told that you have diabetes? How would you tell your mother that she has cancer? How would you tell your aunt and uncle that their six-year-old daughter has just died? Think about these things as you observe your teachers communicating with patients during your training. Some of them will sound like the doctor in the first example noted above; others will be a lot more like the second. I hope you will elect to pattern yourself after the second.

The American Republic will endure until the day Congress discovers that it can bribe the public with the public's money.
—Alexis de Tocqueville

My reading of history convinces me that most bad government results from too much government.
—Thomas Jefferson

Chapter 7

Medical Economics

One day, I walked into the operating room to anesthetize a patient for knee arthroscopy. He was an outpatient, so I had not had an opportunity to see him the night before surgery; however, I knew this man from having taken care of him for his other knee. When he saw me, he smiled broadly and said, "Hey, Doc! How you doing? Say, Doc, I used to wonder why you guys wear those masks in here, and then I got your bill!" Obviously, he was joking with me, and I appreciated the humor immediately; but it does raise the point that medical care costs money.

Unfortunately for you budding physicians, you are unlikely to receive much instruction about medical economics if your institution subscribes to the philosophies of most of the medical schools of my time. Some of the professors in Syracuse took offense at the suggestion that this subject should be broached at all during our training. In their view, medical education was about science, which they taught well. Some told us that if we were interested in learning about business subjects, we should become chiropractors. Looking back over my career, I see that as a narrow and misguided view, one that needs to change. Medicine is a profession, and it is also a business. We need to prepare medical students to be responsible business people and to educate them to join the debate about the financial impact of medical care on society. Because physicians are not properly prepared to exhibit leadership in this arena, others are winning the debate. Those who win, either insurance companies or government, may have only monetary goals in mind, not our patients' welfare. Medical economics is a legitimate subject, and if it is not offered in your curriculum, be certain that you make the effort to educate yourself by reading several of the many books written about it. Please study both capitalist and socialist views of the subject if you wish to develop fully informed opinions, because I do not believe that either side has all the answers. When you have finished your formal training, your specialty society may have continuing education programs dealing with medical economics. Be sure to attend.

It takes money to practice medicine. We have to live, provide for our families, pay off educational debts, and prepare for our retirement. These things require more than apples, chickens, and cheese given in thanks for our efforts. We must buy supplies and equipment, some of which can be astronomically expensive but essential for proper practice. We pay rent or mortgages for offices as well as all the utilities, upkeep, and property taxes. Our nurses, receptionists, technicians, and the numerous other personnel required to run a modern medical practice deserve and demand fair compensation. We must carry professional liability and other insurances to protect us from financial disaster. Finally, never forget that we all pay the government taxes at a dreadfully high rate. If you can tell me how to do all that without money coming in, I would be glad to listen.

So I ask once more: why has it been beneath the dignity of medical schools to teach future physicians about medical economics? Furthermore, why didn't they even suggest that elementary business or economics courses might be fruitful fields of study during our undergraduate years? Now you know in a nutshell why the economics of medical care is so screwed up in this country: most doctors do not know enough about it owing to little or no formal education on the subject. As a result, others who have been so educated drag us around by the nose. This is a critical situation for the future of medicine and one that ought to change. My generation failed to do it, so I hope yours has better luck.

I actually had one lesson in medical economics in medical school, and it came from a strange source. I worked part-time at one of the hospitals in Syracuse during my third and fourth years of medical school. My job was to perform history and physical examinations on patients having specialty surgery the following day, because there were no interns or residents assigned to do those tasks on those services. I did this on average about one or two nights a week. The pay was pretty good, and the extra clinical experience was priceless. One of the surgeons whose patients I often examined was the colorectal surgeon. He was very busy and well-known in the community. Most of my encounters with him were brief and consisted mostly of saying casual but friendly hellos to each other. One evening, he must have been in the mood for conversation, and he started talking to me. He stated quite correctly that they probably were not teaching us much about money in medical school. He reflected for a moment and told me that he had been fully trained and credentialed in colon and rectal surgery. This was news to me, because I had never seen him schedule anything other than rectal procedures like hemorrhoidectomies and pilonidal cystectomies. He told me that the reason he did not do any colon procedures (i.e., intra-abdominal surgery) was that he had been prevented from doing so by the general surgeons of the hospital, who wanted all the intra-abdominal work on the intestinal tract for themselves. I did not know it then, but this is a form of so-called economic credentialing, and it continues today. His reaction to this: "They cut off my legs and laugh because I'm short." It was a poignant but absolutely accurate remark. He then told me where his money went. For each dollar earned, one-third went to run his office, one-third went to the government, and one-third he got to keep. This was an eye-opener for me. I decided on the spot that when I finished my training I would only consider joining practices in which professionals handled the economics, and that is exactly what I did. I subsequently learned that many practitioners would be quite pleased to keep one-third of their gross receipts. That represents the sum total of my medical economics education in medical school.

A license to sell insurance is in some ways a license to steal, in my opinion. I once heard one of the vice presidents of a major insurance company say this in a television interview, "We are a business, not a social program." This, at least, was a truthful statement. The purpose of an insurance company is to make money for its shareholders and especially for its high-echelon executives, all of whom will live in better houses than you will, drive better cars, take more expensive vacations, and send their kids to more expensive schools (whether those schools are better is open to debate). Now all that may be acceptable and, as a dyed-in-the-wool capitalist, I certainly have nothing against making money, but not when it comes through subterfuge instead of merit. Let me first give an example relating to professional liability insurance (I really dislike the term "malpractice insurance"). Back in the 1970s, the multispecialty clinic in the Midwest where I worked paid about $500,000 a year for professional liability coverage for its forty-to-fifty physicians. Suddenly, we were presented with a premium bill for the next year of about $1,500,000. Now it has been a long time since this happened, and the actual amounts might be slightly off but not greatly exaggerated; however, the jump in premium by a factor of about three is accurate. We had done nothing to account for this. In fact, our entire liability history going back to the 1940s was phenomenally good, and we had cost the insurance company nearly nothing compared to what we had paid in premiums over the life of the clinic. The company we dealt with then was one of the industry leaders, but it no longer offers medical professional liability insurance. Because the premium jump was so dramatic, the clinic administrator asked the company to send someone to explain this sudden increase in premiums to our board of directors, of which I was a member at the time. The company complied and sent us an executive who proceeded to tell us that it was not our fault, the whole picture of professional liability was changing, lawsuits were becoming more common, and the amounts of recovery were also going up. We all accepted this as true, because we had been reading some of the same things in the medical literature. I then asked this man if he could tell us how much money in premiums his company took in for professional liability insurance each year and how much they paid out in settlements and jury awards. This was his exact reply: "We don't have those figures." I lied to my father a couple of times during my childhood and suffered the consequences. As a result, I have never appreciated anyone lying to me. If there is one thing insurance companies do well, it is count. I would not be surprised if an insurance company could tell you the average number of hairs on the human thumb, and if there is a significant difference between right and left. They hire brilliant, highly paid mathematicians called actuaries who spend their entire careers crunching numbers so that their executives can keep their big salaries. I told this man that his company had to have that information, and that I was rather angry that he would not share it with us; needless to say, I have had a big problem trusting insurance companies since that evening. If he was telling me the truth, he must have been one of the most poorly informed insurance executives in history.

There are other reasons to mistrust insurance companies and to be upset by their policies. They cheat, hassle, and squeeze in ways that are costly and maddening. Many firms avoid paying claims as long as possible by using a variety of delaying tactics. If they can pay a claim after ninety or one hundred and twenty days instead of thirty, they make quite a bit of interest money. The amount of inconvenience and frustration suffered by patients and health care providers is of no importance to them. I used to get irritated by my own insurance company when I received forms asking if my bout of diverticulitis for which I was hospitalized was work or accident related. Give me a break. This was just an excuse to delay payment to my caregivers. The most exasperating practice of insurance companies, however, is their control over the delivery of care. There are many examples. A simple one involves allowing only thirty days' worth of medicine in a prescription. I understand this as a money-saving policy for the company, but it also causes a lot of inconvenience for the patient. I grant that it is stupid to fill a prescription for six months of a medication, only to have the patient become allergic to it after the third dose. So why not allow only a month's worth or even a week's worth for the first two or three prescriptions and then three months' worth subsequently? My daughter recently tried to fill a prescription for my granddaughter who was suffering from strep throat. The pharmacist told her that the insurance company did not cover that antibiotic, one that is commonly prescribed for that indication. After phone calls to the doctor and the insurance company by the pharmacist, it was learned that the insurance did cover the antibiotic but not in the concentration specified by the doctor. Ridiculous. That sort of harassing of patients, doctors, and pharmacists by insurance companies is simply unacceptable.

A less trivial practice is telling physicians who can and who cannot be allowed in the hospital. I worked with an excellent surgeon, most of whose procedures were done on an outpatient basis. One of his patients had been bleeding quite a bit during the procedure, and the surgeon wanted to observe him in the hospital overnight in case the bleeding should recur. His nurse told him that he would have to call the patient's insurance company to get permission to admit him. This surgeon was known to have a relatively short fuse and could be verbally quite colorful when making a point. I happened to be standing close by when he contacted the representative of his patient's insurance company. He explained the situation clearly and succinctly and said that he would be admitting the patient. She replied that she was terribly sorry, but her company did not allow charges for hospitalization for that procedure. He went ballistic. Wouldn't you? Having first let out a plethora of expletives that would have embarrassed a sailor, he told her quite plainly that she could be the one to explain to the family why the patient had to die if he bled to death at home before being able to return to the hospital. This must have scared her, because he finally got to speak with her supervisor who subsequently approved the admission. The whole incident should not have happened. It should clearly have been the surgeon's call to admit or not admit, not the insurance company's. Tragically, this kind of thing gets worse all the time, and it will be and already is insufferable under government control.

If you do not believe me about medicine being insufferable under government control, perhaps this story will change your mind. Early one Saturday morning, a woman was admitted to the hospital having been stabbed by her daughter's boyfriend. She had thirty-seven distinct stab wounds in the chest and abdomen and was in extremis when she arrived at the hospital, where she was taken urgently to the operating room for exploration. She had lost a lot of blood. The anesthesiologist who had been on call on Friday night came in first and, on seeing the severity of the patient's injuries, he recognized that she would be in surgery for a long time. He decided to bring in the anesthesiologist on call for Saturday rather than summoning a nurse anesthetist for help. The two of them stayed with the patient during surgery. She needed a lot of blood, and it would have been virtually impossible for one individual alone to keep up with her blood replacement and other care during the surgery that lasted for many hours. Both the anesthesia and surgical teams worked incredibly hard. Although she survived to be taken to the intensive care unit, she ultimately required more surgery and, in the end, she died. When all was said and done, the two anesthesiologists submitted bills to Medicaid for their services, although the second anesthesiologist's bill was significantly less than the one the primary anesthesiologist submitted. Medicaid refused to pay for the second anesthesiologist. They argued that a paramedic, nurse, or anyone else would have been enough help under the circumstances. Even though I had not been involved in the case, I was livid. I insisted that the second anesthesiologist resubmit his bill. He did, and it was rejected once again. I suggested that he demand a face-to-face meeting to protest the rejection, but he opted not to do that. Now if you were lying near death on an operating table with thirty-seven holes in you and required extraordinary care, would you prefer to have two anesthesiologists or an anesthesiologist and an untrained helper? So be it for the fairness of government medicine. The only thing important to the government is the bottom line.

You merely have to watch television and read the newspapers a little to learn of other insurance company practices that drive physicians and patients crazy. For one thing, because of their primary profit motive, they do not want to insure the sick. Now I can understand having a problem insuring someone who has electively gone bare for some time and who now applies for insurance because he has developed diabetes. I have a harder time understanding why someone with a long-standing but stable condition, such as depression, who is now healthy, can be refused insurance, not just for psychiatric conditions but for all illnesses. Insurance companies may also refuse to cover new or experimental treatments of common diseases, such as breast cancer, where new treatments may have the best chance of helping the patient. There are problems that the public does not understand about this particular dilemma, in that some experimental treatments are incredibly expensive making the insurance companies less likely to cover them. So why can't the company offer you an option up front, before you get sick, for coverage of new and experimental treatments even if that option carries a slight rise in premiums?

I certainly do not have the answers as to how medicine should be financed; however, from what I have observed, neither does anyone else. If anyone out there has the answer, please speak up, but don't just say, "Let the government do it." If you do not want your government to do your grocery shopping or house hunting for you, for goodness sake, do not let them get control of your medical care. How do we determine fair values for new procedures, equipment, and drugs? How do we adjust fees for geographical differences? While capitalism and the free market have classically been allowed to determine most of these things, it is possible that some form of regulated capitalism will have to be employed in the future to pay for medical care. We must be certain, however, that the regulation does not come strictly from the government. No matter the cost, we cannot afford to let the government control the practice of medicine. Furthermore, insurance companies ought to have less say in the control of medical care. To be fair, I also believe that outlier medical practitioners who try to milk any system ought to start losing their licenses. Completely socialized medicine is an undesirable alternative for patients, for doctors, and for the continuing development of medical technology. Citizens may perceive socialized medicine as wonderful because they see it as "free," but nothing as complex and expensive as medical care is free. Think for a moment what kind of car you would get if the government decided to provide everyone with an automobile and forbid you from making your own choice. You can bet the car would more likely resemble a Yugo than a Lamborghini, unless, of course, you were president or senator! The same is true of socialized medicine, because the most important thing to the government is the bottom line. Elected officials have so many self-interests that they cannot be trusted with something as important as our health care, an unfortunate but accurate assessment in my opinion. They are so politically motivated they cannot examine the issues in an unbiased fashion. If you cannot recognize the truth of that, you have not observed our political process long enough. Politicians at the highest levels seek only three things: power, money, and reelection. We should not allow those three things to influence our medical care.

Lest I appear overly cynical about our government, allow me to share a bit of my political philosophy with you. We live in America, and we cherish freedom. Complete freedom, of course, is impossible because it implies the absence of consequences or responsibility. Humans learned centuries ago that complete freedom does not work whenever two or more of us are gathered in the same place, so governments were devised in part to codify which freedoms were acceptable and which were not. Our current meaning of freedom is really that of freedom to choose and is more or less based on the premise that where one person's freedom ends, another's begins. The beauty of our Constitution is that it allows us so many choices. I believe government per se is abhorrent to the human being, because none of us likes to be told what to do and to have someone watching us to make sure that we do it. The word "government" means to control and manage and ought to be a detestable term to an intelligent, freedom-loving, honest individual. George Washington may have said it best: "Government is not reason; it is not eloquent; it is force. Like fire, it is a dangerous servant and a fearful master." Ronald Reagan waggishly stated, "Government is not a solution to our problem, government is the problem." The trick is to have just enough government so that we can all enjoy the most fundamental freedoms, choices, and protections. We must recognize that each time we relinquish a choice to the government, we give up some of our freedom. This, of course, includes asking the government to do for us what we can do very well for ourselves.

I hope you will agree that ours is not a perfect government, nor is any other. We have been more or less civilized for over eight thousand years, and yet there has been no perfect government designed in that time. Perhaps there is a message in that incredible and glaring failure. I believe it can be blamed on the fundamental mendacity of mankind. The word "mendacity" implies lying; but in my mind, it also implies deceit, treachery, hypocrisy, selfishness, and subterfuge. Having observed and contemplated the actions of politicians in a variety of nations for more than half a century, I believe that many of them have elevated mendacity to a fine art and regularly practice it. Achieving high office either by election or force is a difficult and dirty business, which means that many who rise to the top are likely to be the most mendacious (and dangerous) of all. This prevents governments from being truly open, fair, impartial, honest, and altruistic, because governments are largely composed of individuals who are most concerned with their own selfish interests and not those of the people they supposedly serve. Those who govern profess to have all the answers and force their wills on the populace either with bullets or taxes and regulations. I hasten to accuse both liberal and conservative politicians of being guilty of the behaviors I have just described. Mendacity is emphatically bipartisan. As a result, I am totally suspicious of all governments and wish to have no more of their intrusion into my life than absolutely necessary. Those, incidentally, were the views of the majority of our founding fathers in America, and it appears that one has to be cautious about agreeing with them nowadays. Charles Austin Beard, an American historian who died in 1948, wrote, "You need only reflect that one of the best ways to get yourself a reputation as a dangerous citizen these days is to go about repeating the very phrases which our founding fathers used in the struggle for independence." His statement certainly seems relevant today. This is the age of "political correctness," and if you think that you truly have freedom of speech, you are sadly mistaken. These are my opinions and observations of government; if they are viewed as cynical, so be it.

We need to find some way for health care providers, equipment and drug manufacturers, hospitals and clinics, insurance companies, and consumers to come together to attack the problems of paying for medical care without the heavy hand of government interfering. One of our problems is that we never hear real data about the costs of providing the best medical care in the world. We only hear demagogues telling us that hospitals charge too much, doctors charge too much, and too many people cannot afford insurance. Good medical care is costly! The marvelous imaging devices that have helped save so many lives and alleviate so much suffering cost at least seven figures each and need to be regularly replaced to keep up with the improving technology. Do we want to abandon those machines and the technological improvements? To have realistic solutions, we need realistic information. It is long overdue for us to approach this problem in a rational and nonpolitical way. I hope your generation can get the job done.

I do not want you to get any wrong ideas from what I have written about insurance companies, government, and medical economics. I have lived a comfortable life financially and otherwise. I am quite aware that the checks have primarily come from insurance companies and the government on behalf of my patients, and I am very grateful. I have no complaints about what I have earned, and I am well aware that I could have earned a lot more in another profession. I have worked hard and been rewarded appropriately in my opinion. Many anesthesiologists these days earn well over $300,000 per year. I never reached that figure. I can say that during my practice lifetime, even though I had regular raises during the first twenty years, my buying power never exceeded the buying power of my salary in 1974 when I became a partner in the clinic in Iowa. In essence, I did not earn more money over the years but simply kept up with inflation, something for which I am most thankful. Certainly we are paid well, even after paying a third or more of it in taxes, and much of my time in practice occurred during the years of 50 percent federal rates; however, in view of what we must do to earn it, I do not think our financial compensation is outlandish. Money for doctors is not my highest concern. I am confident that doctors and other health care professionals are always going to be paid reasonably well; otherwise, there will not be many providers that people would be willing to trust with their lives. To do what we do, you must be intelligent, well educated, dedicated, willing to work exceptionally hard, and have the stomach to do things that most human beings could not or would not do. For the most part, people with those qualifications are not going to be happy working for peanuts.

I am most concerned about the control of health care. There are two golden rules. The first states that we should treat others as we would like to be treated ourselves. The second golden rule reminds us of this simple truth: "He who has the gold makes the rules!" Back in the Clinton administration, there was a huge battle over the control of health care. Was it going to be the health care industry itself (physicians, hospitals, drug companies, etc.), the insurance industry, or government? The insurance industry won out. With the Obama administration, the government won out and it did so in an especially heinous, heavy-handed fashion, in the opinions of many people, including me. This was done first and foremost, because the politicians at the highest levels wanted control of the 16 percent or so of the U.S. economy represented by health care. They want you dependent on them, and what better way to ensure your dependency than to take control of your health care. The problem with the government being at the reins is that the most important considerations are control and the bottom line. I know that is repetitive of me, but it cannot be said enough, so you will probably hear it again. Major advances in medicine will not come as regularly as they do now and delivery of care will suffer. The government will claim that it will not allow rationing of care, but that is exactly what it will do. The march toward total control of medical care by the government has begun. It will be nearly impossible to turn it back, and, while it may start slowly, it will surge at light speed before anyone realizes what a major mistake we have made. Try to remember that statement one day when you treat a patient in a rational, successful manner and learn that the government refuses to pay you because it was not an approved treatment in their book. Remember it when the government approves only four antibiotics for a condition, but your patient is allergic to all four and cannot afford to pay for options five or six. By the way, some of this is already happening with insurance companies, those entities whose admitted raison d'être is precisely to make money. The government will be much worse, because the government always tries to make everything "one size fits all." It is too bad that people just do not come in one size, especially with regard to their medical care needs.

Sound pessimistic? I urge you to read about the health care systems in other countries. An excellent place to start reading is a book by T. R. Reid entitled *The Healing of America: A Global Quest for Better, Cheaper, and Fairer Health Care* (Penguin Press, New York, 2009). Mr. Reid went around the world experiencing a variety of health care systems and wrote about them in detail. Some systems are not bad, while others are frightening. I am distressed that our government did not closely and publicly examine other systems in the world and try to fashion the recent health care legislation to incorporate the best of all of them, some of which are based on cooperation between government and free enterprise. They chose instead to do their debating in a one-sided, closed-door, back-room manner. Judging from former Speaker of the House Nancy Pelosi's statement that we will find out what is in the health care bill when they pass it, our system is headed toward becoming an alarming disaster that will be deaf to the cries of the people. That kind of arrogance from one of the country's most powerful legislators is appalling and flies in the face of everything I was taught about American freedom. I went through the original one-thousand-page House bill. It was both difficult and scary. The words were technically English, but the bill was written in such an arcane fashion as to be meaningless to the average citizen. Only the creation of a new and draconian bureaucracy came through in vivid detail. It was especially disturbing to me that the appointment of members to that bureaucracy seemed to be based more on the political correctness of the appointee rather than on competence. What other forms of arrogance and control lay ahead? This worries me a great deal, much more than any changes in physician compensation. It should worry both you and your future patients.

You will be impressed as you begin your future in clinical medicine with how much waste is generated simply by having to follow harsh and unreasonable regulations. We have recently been saddled with regulations aimed at preventing infections but which are so wasteful as to be shameful. We will throw away millions and millions of dollars worth of drugs every year due to these regulations and for nothing. In twenty years of taking care of ophthalmic surgery patients (now approaching thirty thousand patients), I have not caused a single infection. Others practicing my subspecialty have had exactly the same experience, and it is safe to say that millions of patients have been managed in a way that did not lead to infection. We are now being told, however, that the way we have done things in drawing up our drugs prior to administration is not good enough, and we must do as we are told or suffer significant consequences. It is their way or the highway, as the saying goes. If none of us have had any infections, what the hell are we going to prevent? We are going to prevent the system from being solvent, that's what!

Another incredibly wasteful exercise in medicine is the medical record. The record used to be measured in pages. Thanks to regulatory and survey agencies that require so many different levels and types of documentation, the medical record is now measured in pounds. All this, of course, was designed to improve care. It has made it worse! It certainly has not reduced the number of lawsuits. Treating the medical record is expensive and unbelievably time consuming. Nurses now spend more time at the nursing station filling out papers or working at computers than they do administering to the sick. It is horrifying, dangerous, and sad. I was hospitalized in Illinois a few years ago with acute diverticulitis. For two days, I did not have a clean set of sheets, a clean hospital gown, nor a bath, all the while feeling terrible and being horribly diaphoretic because of my fever. I literally had no care except for the taking of my vital signs every six hours and the administration of my intravenous antibiotic, a once-a-day encounter. Not trying to sound like a snob, I would point out that I am a doctor. You would think that they would have bent over backward to give me good care. The opposite was the case. I am not blaming the nurses. Other forces compel them to comply with these well-meaning but onerous record-keeping regulations. When I was an orderly before starting medical school, we gave each patient a bath every morning, again later in the day if needed, and kept the bed linens fresh and clean as often as required. Patients also received a back rub every morning and night. I am reminded of a story told many years ago by a wonderful, gentle comedian named Sam Levenson. On a television program, Sam told the story of himself and his wife dealing with a crying baby. They got out their copy of Dr. Spock's baby book and began thumbing through the pages. As the baby bawled, they ticked off all the possibilities: has the baby been fed, does the baby have a fever, is the baby clean and dry, is the baby's diaper too tight, does the baby have a rash, and so on. In each instance, they were certain that everything was just fine. As they stood by the crib deeply concentrating on the book with the baby lying there shrieking louder than ever, the baby's grandmother came into the nursery and picked him up out of the crib with a loving hug. The baby instantly quieted. In our hospitals, thanks to expensive and wasteful regulations and inappropriate demands on our nurses, the babies will keep right on crying for the foreseeable future.

It is unfair to simply employ criticism or cynicism when attacking any problem, so I ought to offer some constructive comments about all this. While I may not be smart enough to come up with the ultimate solution to the financing of health care, I do know that we must be certain to address several key issues in any system we adopt. Here are some of them:

1. There needs to be an open, honest, and thorough national discussion in this country as to whether health care is a right. It is not specified as such in the Constitution, and I am personally unaware of any body of law in our country that defines health care as a right of all individuals.

After the debate, perhaps we should have a plebiscite on the issue to settle it. As it is now, we have one party saying it is and the other saying it is not. I think each of us has the right to make this decision. If it is determined by popular vote that health care is a right, then we need to forge ahead to see how we can best finance it.

2. It is essential to maintain the freedom to choose your own doctor at any time. Our government is likely to restrict this choice if certain models already in place are followed. They might say that you are free to choose—once a year. This is unacceptable. We are a free people, and freedom to choose our own health care providers should be nonnegotiable. We ought to be able to choose the doctors and facilities best suited for the management of our specific medical problems. If those doctors and facilities happen to be in another city or another state, the coverage should still be provided. The same freedom to choose ought to be extended to our insurance companies. If the company insuring us does not live up to its promises, we should have the right to find one that will. We must not accept anything less, because anything less is simply tyranny and totally inappropriate in this or any country.

3. Everyone should be covered. If an insurance-based system is adopted, anyone able to pay the premium should be accepted for coverage. Those unable to pay the premium may have to be covered by the government. Exclusions because of illness are unacceptable.

4. There ought to be a standard policy that covers all the common ailments and treatments, including trauma. In some systems, coverage for things, such as cosmetic plastic surgery, experimental treatments, and others can be purchased separately by the individual. A combination of government and private financing can work and, in my view, ought to be investigated more thoroughly.

5. Decisions about medical care must be left to the health care professionals and their patients. I do not object to stringent laws and punishments for unscrupulous practitioners who try to cheat the system, but the rest of us should be left free to make our decisions based on the needs of our patients and not the decrees written in a government proclamation. Control of your care by the government is one of the most sinister aspects of socialized medicine. We must not let it happen. There were no students named "Government" or "Insurance" in my medical school class, and I will bet there are not any in yours, either.

6. The cost of medical care must not become a line item in the national budget. We cannot ration medical care in this way. We need what we need. We can have a discussion about what entities and treatments ought to be included in the standard policy. We can have a discussion about the costs of providing care. In the end, however, the cost of providing medical care cannot be reduced to a predetermined slice in the pie chart of the government's budget.
7. A co-payment of some kind must accompany all care. This is necessary to prevent abuse of the system by those who would use it inappropriately for every sniffle and scratch. The co-payment might differ from illness to illness, and I would suggest it be higher for minor ailments than for major. It might also be means tested, being significantly less for those having low incomes.
8. There needs to be a major change in medical-legal issues in this country. Please see the chapter of the same name in this book for some suggestions. The change also needs to address the pharmaceutical and medical device industries that face huge class-action lawsuits when unexpected issues arise after their products are approved and put on the market. It is naïve and disingenuous to aver that the cost of medical care is not significantly affected by the current medical-legal climate.
9. Any system proposed must address funding for education and research, both of which are costly but offer the only real means of advancing medical science and patient care.
10. We must also provide for maintenance of health care facilities and technological improvements. There is a lot more to the cost of medical care than salaries for doctors and nurses. We cannot ignore these essential components.

I hope I have convinced you that I have applied some rational thinking to the problems of medical economics and not just spewed criticism and cynicism. As already noted, I do not have all the answers, but I find it difficult to accept any system in which a government as imperfect as ours is in complete control of medical care and financing. To solve the problems, we need a long, thorough, honest national debate. The process we just came through with Mr. Obama and the Democrat Congress was anything but a national debate. It was a railroad job performed with the lights off. Not only do we deserve better than that, I am convinced we can and will do better.

I will cut this chapter short with just a few more comments. First of all, never be embarrassed about submitting a bill for your care of the patient. You work hard, you provide essential services, and you deserve to be fairly compensated for it. If the plumber, electrician, and carpenter deserve to be paid, so does the doctor and all health care providers. If it is expected that you pay the car dealer for your new car, the dealer should be expected to pay you for removing his diseased appendix and saving his life. Second, never charge more than you are entitled to receive. Send a complete and honest bill for what you have done and be able to document it. It is unethical and, in most instances, illegal to do otherwise. It is also unnecessary to do otherwise. There is plenty of disease to go around, and you will be busy. You ought to be able to make enough money to meet your needs without cheating. Third, if you are entering medicine to be filthy rich, you have made a mistake. You will be comfortable, but the real money in this country is made in corporate boardrooms, on Wall Street, in Hollywood, on sporting fields, and in other bastions of capitalism (the greatest economic system on the planet). You are entering a service industry and will become a well-paid servant of the people. Accept that and be happy in what you do while praying that it will not be an insurance company or the government telling you how to do it. Finally, remember always that in the practice of medicine, the bottom line is the patient's welfare. If you remember that, you will not have any trouble achieving modest financial success. Your greatest achievement, however, ought to be your satisfaction in having helped a fellow human being.

We have the means to change the laws we find unjust or onerous. We cannot, as citizens, pick and choose the laws we will or will not obey.
—Ronald Reagan

Chapter 8

Know the Rules and Obey Them

Life is filled with rules. You have been a student all your life and have been exposed to many. Do not think that you will escape them after finishing your training, because, if anything, the rules just get tougher, grow more demanding, and carry bigger consequences if you do not follow them. My purposes in this chapter are to talk a little bit about rules in general, to give some examples of times when I have observed them being broken, and to leave you feeling that life is better and easier if you live by the rules.

I pause to explain that the regulations I will be talking about are not like those in poetry, art, philosophy, science, or design. There are rules in these disciplines to be sure; but the most memorable practitioners are the ones who severely stretched, broke, or rewrote them. This chapter will be oriented toward the behavioral guidelines that govern our personal interactions, rules that are more codified than those just mentioned and that include both etiquette and law. Remember, policies that address behavior are the constructs of the human mind and are, thus, subject to amendment, refinement, and even revocation. Be cautioned, however, that it takes a brave and determined person to initiate the forces to accomplish those changes.

Civilization could not exist without laws. Anarchy is chaos, especially with so many of us aboard this old planet. These things being so, it has continually bothered me that certain individuals among us get their jollies by defying the rules. I do not want you to think that I am a goody-two-shoes without guilt in this area, because, like almost everyone else, I tested, ignored, and even broke a few rules during my developing years. That is not something I am particularly proud of, mind you, and I am glad I got it out of my system at an early age and realized that life is a whole lot simpler if you do your best to follow the rules. You should have determined that for yourself by now too. One of my classmates in our first year of medical school cheated all semester long in physiology before being turned in for cheating by twelve different students during the final exam. My uncle was in seminary at the same time, and when I told him about this incident, he informed me that three of his classmates had been caught cheating. I was appalled that my classmate was given another chance and allowed to repeat the first year by joining the class behind us. In my opinion, he should have been old enough and wise enough not to cheat and should have been summarily tossed out. There was no doubt of his guilt. Cheating is juvenile, unacceptable behavior and should not exist beyond kindergarten. Do not be tempted to cheat, because when you do, the real victims are your patients; and if you have any conscience at all, you will become a victim of your own guilt at some point.

You would think that only the knuckle draggers of society would ignore the rules, but the opposite seems to be the case. The intelligent seem to find extreme delight in bending or breaking the law. The name Bernie Madoff immediately comes to mind. In case you have just arrived on planet Earth, Bernie Madoff is a man who was convicted of bilking a whole bunch of people out of an enormous amount of money in a Ponzi scheme. As he was intelligent and successful, why would he feel compelled to do such a thing? I doubt that we will ever know for certain. Perhaps the greedy and cunning areas of his cerebral cortex overpowered the rational and moral areas, wherever all those are and assuming he has any moral areas at all. He obviously was not the first in history to be so greedy and mendacious, but he does stand out as a warning for us all. You may break the rules in dozens of ways in multiple areas and get away with minor or insignificant penalties, but those caught with a hand in the cash register suffer the entire weight of the legal system, just as surely as they hung horse thieves in the old days. That is a solid fact and one to remember.

Society does not expect physicians or other health care professionals to be lawbreakers, and we are often held to standards well above those used to judge others; thus, we are constantly subject to the scrutiny of our peers and society as a whole. In fact, an argument can be made that we are more critically viewed than many others in our society. I believe this is entirely fitting and proper because ours is a profession that demands honesty, fair play, and selflessness. If you disagree with that, please stop reading and go find yourself another profession, perhaps politics. Witnessing someone intentionally breaking the rules is painful, especially if doing so is not in the best interest of the patient.

One of the most egregious cases of rule-breaking that I have personally witnessed occurred one night when I was on call. It was late, and I was about to go to bed when the phone rang. I hoped that the call did not mean that I would have to go in for surgery, but the results of the call gave me anything but a good night's sleep. It was the nursing supervisor at the hospital who was in charge for that evening, and she told me that an orthopedic surgeon, the one I have already mentioned as being terribly truculent, had just ordered a patient to receive a unit of blood. The problem was that this patient, well-known to me, was a Jehovah's Witness and had made it clear from the get-go that she did not want anything to do with blood or blood products. When the nurse reminded the surgeon of this, he bluntly told her that it did not make any difference to him. He firmly insisted that she be given the blood and that the nurse must do anything she could to disguise the blood, including wrapping it in aluminum foil or her pantyhose if necessary. This nurse was both intelligent and experienced and had no intention of carrying out such an absurd order. She also knew that this surgeon was an exception to the others on staff and was a chronic problem in many areas. She called me because I was on call and because I had anesthetized the patient for her surgery earlier in the day. I had seen the patient in the late afternoon and had noted her postoperative blood count, which was quite acceptable. There was no indication for the transfusion based on that laboratory finding, and in addition, the patient was quite well clinically. This surgeon was an interesting study. He had practiced for many years, was skilled in his work, had a loyal following in the community and among his peers, could at times charm the scales off a snake, had a drinking problem, and had an ego beyond belief. To this day, I believe that he ordered the blood because he was not going to have some mere patient tell him what he could and could not do. In ordering the blood, he was ordering a criminal assault on the patient, an act that is not only unethical but also clearly illegal. The patient did not receive the blood, recovered fully, and went home.

Even though I was the most junior partner in our clinic at that time and he was one of the most senior, I initiated charges for dismissal against this surgeon. I presented the charges to the entire partnership group in his presence. He did not say a word in his defense. There were no impassioned pleas for or against him, although several voiced their displeasure that he would do something so outrageous. There were thirty voting partners at that time, and the final vote was fifteen to dismiss and fifteen to retain. It required a majority to dismiss. I was shocked by the result, and it bothers me even now that fifteen physicians would vote to retain a man guilty of ordering an assault on a patient. One of the senior partners told me that he could not vote against this man because he had been so important in the care of one of his family members. That did not impress me. I would have voted against my father or one of my own children had they ordered an assault on a patient.

I was disappointed by the vote both because of the seriousness of this man's actions in this case and because he was a problem in so many other ways. Life goes on, however, and the next day was a busy one, which helped to take my mind off my defeat. Several of my younger colleagues commiserated and assured me that when they became partners, the outcome would be totally different. At the end of the day, I drove home and pulled the car into the garage. Taped to the door leading into the house was a large poster showing a kitten looking very distressed while dangling from a small tree branch by its forepaws. The caption in big bold letters read, "Hang in there, baby!" My dear wife succeeded in easing my pain with humor.

The surgeon kept a low profile for a while, but ultimately his abnormal behavior patterns surfaced again, and he was finally dismissed by a wide margin on a matter of ethics involving an inappropriate sexual innuendo to a patient. I relate this case of his ordering an illegal action to illustrate that physicians are capable of breaking the rules and that sometimes the consequences are not what they should be. Had the nurses followed his orders, I suspect that he would have been subject to criminal charges and may well have gone to jail, although the nurses would also have been in big trouble for carrying out such an order. Lawyers criticize us for not policing ourselves. Here is an instance in which they were correct, even though we got around to doing the right thing in the end. I can only say that when someone is breaking the rules for other than the patient's best interest, that person should be challenged as thoroughly as possible. A nurse should never carry out an order that is clearly illegal or unethical and should report such an order immediately to someone who is trustworthy and who can see that appropriate action is taken.

Are there legitimate reasons to break the rules? The answer is yes, if it is obviously and arguably in the best interest of the patient. Suppose for a moment that you work in a surgery center dedicated to ophthalmology that has a firm policy of starting no surgery after 4:00 p.m., with the expectation that all patients will have been discharged by 5:30 p.m. to avoid paying overtime to the staff involved in the patients' care. Today a patient presents at 4:25 p.m. with a retinal condition that requires urgent surgical treatment to salvage any hope of retaining vision. What do you do? You keep the surgery center open and do the surgery. You pay overtime to the staff willing to stay on, and you ignore the policy. Why? Doing so is in the best interest of the patient. We exist and do what we do for the best interest of our patients. This is precisely what is dangerous about government medicine. Not only would the government be disinclined to pay for surgery done under such circumstances, it might actually penalize those who ignored the policy. Why? To the government, it is the policy (i.e., control) that is important, not the patient. Rules are rules, but sometimes they need to be ignored to do the right thing. The trick is to learn when it is proper and permissible to ignore them and to learn which ones can be bent or broken for the benefit of the patient without serious consequences to yourself or others.

The rules of our society are based loosely on the Roman model. In ancient Rome, there were two kinds of laws: *mores* and *leges*. Our terms moral, immoral, legal, illegal and many others come from these roots. Mores were those codes of behavior that were not necessarily written down but were universally recognized as defining proper, virtuous behavior. Mores were extremely important to the Romans and dealt with matters of deportment, personal behavior, and civility—things we regard as moral behavior and etiquette. Mores were held in such high regard that Roman citizens were loath to disregard them for fear of the reactions of their fellow citizens, such as being ostracized. Leges were the written laws decreed by the senate and/or emperor and might carry severe punishment by the state if broken. The same general scheme of things survives to this day, and we continue to make distinctions between behaviors that are strictly immoral versus those that are strictly illegal, although there certainly is blending between the two.

As a health care professional, you will be held to both moral and legal standards. We will talk more about moral standards in other chapters. Legal standards come from a variety of sources, including federal, state, and local statutes as well as hospital and clinic bylaws. People tend to fear the federal, state, and local statutes because of their obvious severe penalties, but you must be equally mindful of the hospital and clinic bylaws because they will be the rules that have the greatest impact on your daily behavior. Disregarding the hospital and clinic policies can have serious consequences, including loss of privileges, loss of income, and even dismissal. One good thing about bylaws is that you can amend them if you can convince enough people to agree with you that a change is needed. It is exceedingly difficult to alter federal, state, or local statutes, but you can arouse the citizenry if you have the energy and will.

The threat of losing one's hospital privileges is a classic way in which bylaws are enforced against physicians. At the hospital I practiced in for many years, there was a policy that required you to attend the monthly medical staff meetings. If you are anything like me, I suspect that you are going to find that meetings and committee assignments are among the biggest pains in the butt forced on you in medicine; nonetheless, they have a purpose and, on balance, do more good than harm. At this hospital, if you missed more than three meetings, you were supposed to lose your privileges. The hospital tried to make the meeting attractive by giving us dinner, making it as much a social affair as a business and educational gathering. This was not average hospital fare. The dietary staff outdid themselves and gave us great meals. You could be excused if you were on call and working or if you happened to be out of town. One of the practitioners in town chronically blew off these meetings. I do not know if he suffered agoraphobia or simply did not want someone else telling him what to do. I suspect it was a lot more of the latter than the former. Anyway, after sending him multiple warnings that he would lose his privileges if he did not attend, the medical staff, in its collective wisdom, changed the bylaws so that you could miss four meetings. Then they changed them again so that you could miss six. This was a classic case of the tail wagging the dog. Because it was a city-owned hospital, the medical staff knew that if they pulled his privileges, it would be all over the front page of the newspaper; therefore, instead of doing the right thing, they changed the bylaws to try and comply with his behavior. That was nuts. He still did not obey the rule. My advice: if you have a good rule, one followed by nearly everyone, never change it for an outlier, even if it means headlines in the local paper. Sometimes headlines are a bigger threat to the culprit than loss of privileges.

Another way to lose one's privileges is to get too far behind in paperwork. Physician's paperwork for the most part involves dictating operative notes (which ought to be done right after surgery in the first place), discharge summaries, histories and physicals (which should be done within twenty-four hours of admission), and progress notes (a daily task). It also includes signing verbal orders, the face sheet, and all dictated notes. Nurses and other health care personnel pretty much do their paperwork on a shift-by-shift basis and avoid getting behind. When we were interns and residents, they had a great way of insuring that we kept up with our paperwork: you were not allowed to take vacation if your paperwork was not up to date, and if you did, you would be fired when you returned. Why all the fuss about paperwork? If the paperwork is not complete, the hospital cannot bill for its services; so if you are sixty days behind in signing your charts, the hospital is that far behind in billing. If all the staff members are sixty days behind, it spells financial disaster for the hospital. You can take my word for it that you will lose your privileges much faster for being behind in record keeping than you will if you neglect going to staff meetings. Both are important things to do, but skipping the meeting does not affect the bottom line. Have I ever seen anyone lose hospital privileges? You bet! It is usually a temporary loss until the paperwork is completed, but in some cases, a monetary penalty is also imposed. The moral of the story: obey the bylaws and, you will keep your privileges.

I have another interesting story about hospital privileges. You will remember the surgeon I told you about earlier who tried to transfuse a Jehovah's Witness. When we finally fired him from our clinic, he still had hospital privileges and could have set up an independent practice in town and continued to operate. Shortly after we had fired him, it came time for all of us to renew our hospital privileges, an annual or biennial chore I know you are going to enjoy. We all got notices from the hospital with the appropriate forms to fill in and everyone complied as usual—except him. The hospital sent him several notices as required by the bylaws, including copies of the appropriate articles in the bylaws dealing with this issue. The final notice was sent by registered mail with a return receipt and included the warning, as had the others, that failure to comply would result in complete loss of privileges. The required time lapsed without his responding, so the hospital sent him a notice that his privileges were withdrawn. He sued the hospital and the members of the medical staff executive committee who were all members of our clinic. In most instances, the law does not look kindly upon interfering with one's livelihood, so we were a bit nervous, even though the hospital had done everything exactly right according to the bylaws. We had no intention of backing down from the lawsuit, but we did wonder where the money would come from if he won the suit. We approached our professional liability insurance company to ask if this sort of thing was covered by our policy. After examining all the facts, the company's attorney met with us and informed us that the company would indeed cover us. They felt that we had done everything correctly, and, in the case of this particular practitioner, they felt that we had served the public well in addition. It was one time when I felt especially proud of and thankful for an insurance company. The lawsuit was dropped, and so far as I know, he never practiced in that hospital again.

Many rules can be broken resulting in a variety of consequences. In one of the subspecialties of our clinic, there were two practitioners, Dr. A and Dr. B. Dr. A had been there longer and was a difficult man to deal with due to a huge ego and sense of self-importance, but he was brilliant and did his job well. His nurse was also a difficult person to work with and had a frightful reputation within the clinic for being fractious, bossy, and sometimes downright nasty. There was always a bit of friction between Dr. A and Dr. B based on differences of opinions as well as differences in personalities. One day, Dr. A's nurse, in a fit of temper (her most common state of being), called Dr. B a son of a bitch in front of several people. I do not remember for sure if it was just in front of other staff members or if there were patients present, but it makes little difference. In the first place, Dr. B was not a son of a bitch, was very good at his specialty, and was well liked by virtually everyone in the clinic. In the second place, insubordination of this degree is generally not tolerated in any workplace. The clinic's administrator, upon hearing of the incident, investigated to be certain it had happened and then fired her that day. Dr. A was furious that his nurse had been canned, and he immediately went to the board of directors of the clinic to complain. I had just begun my second tour of duty on the board when this happened. Dr. A appeared before the committee and announced that if we did not rehire his nurse at once, he would leave. Some of the other members of the committee seemed worried that Dr. A would leave if we did not rehire the nurse, resulting in a big gap in care. Both of these specialists were quite busy. The rest of us were shocked that anyone would be willing to accede to his demand. We argued that it was unconscionable that Dr. A dared to blackmail us by threatening to leave. We further argued that Dr. B was not a son of a bitch, that the nurse was a chronic pain in everybody's neck and had been so for years, that rehiring her would cause our administrator to lose face and totally undermine his authority, and that rehiring her would send the message that it is acceptable to call one of the bosses a son of a bitch (i.e., insubordination is permissible). The board refused to rehire her, and Dr. A left. In short order, we hired Dr. C, who got along famously with everyone, was excellent in his specialty, and was an asset to the clinic and the community. The moral of this story: never fall for blackmail. Life is like sticking your thumb in a bucket of water. You make an impression for a while, but when the thumb is removed, the gap is instantly filled. No one is irreplaceable. If your ego is over the moon, you will never believe that, but it is true nevertheless.

Rules can be broken by nearly anyone working in a hospital or clinic. There was a period of time when the OR nurses in our hospital complained of losing money from their purses when they came in for emergency cases. Nothing ever seemed to be taken during the day, just at night. The nursing administrators did some excellent detective work to solve the mystery. The thefts were documented by date. They never involved the same OR nurses, the same surgeons or surgeons' nurses, nor the same anesthesia staff; but they almost always occurred when the emergency cases involved general surgery or orthopedics. It was then determined that the thefts uniformly occurred when an X-ray was required during surgery, from which they were able to determine that the same X-ray technician was present each time there was a theft. The nurses approached the chief radiology technician who told them that they had just begun to notice thefts from the lockers in the radiology department. They went to the police, who provided them with money that had been marked with an invisible substance that became visible under ultraviolet light. The money came up missing, and the suspected X-ray technician was confronted. She immediately denied everything and refused examination with the ultraviolet light. She immediately disappeared, never to be seen again, and the stealing stopped. One important lesson learned is that if everyone is honest, bad things like this will not happen. Unfortunately, you cannot count on everyone being honest. The second lesson is that good record keeping makes for good detective work, so keep good records.

You get into serious trouble if you mess with the feds, and I have never understood how someone could willingly and knowingly defraud the government by billing Medicaid and Medicare more than what they are entitled to receive. If the feds suspect you of fraud, I have been told that they storm into your office unannounced and armed, then seal all your records and confiscate them. They effectively shut you down while they perform their investigation, and you stay that way until you prove your innocence, pay a humongous fine, or go to jail. I once read a newspaper article about a fraudulent practitioner. His office was in a poorer neighborhood. This guy (I refuse to call him a physician despite his credentials) sat behind his desk all day while patients filtered in and sat down before him. His only question: "What do you want today?" He would then write out a prescription, give it to the patient, and bill Medicaid or Medicare as if he had done a full examination. Without ever touching a patient, he wrote out prescriptions for all kinds of medications, including barbiturates, opioids, and other controlled substances. In some instances, those drugs were then sold on the open market by the persons he had given the prescriptions. In my view, this foul individual needed to lose his license and do serious jail time. He was not a physician; he was simply a drug dealer with a degree. His practice was illegal and unethical, and it bothers me terribly that his was not an isolated case. There are all kinds of ways to defraud Medicaid and Medicare, and there are many people out there doing it, not all of them physicians. Purveyors of medical supplies also have opportunities to defraud, and some of them do. Do not aid and abet the defrauding of anyone. If you seriously suspect fraud, get your ducks in a row with solid evidence before turning anyone in to the authorities. Investigation of fraud is a painful and potentially destructive business. Never turn anyone in without proper, incontrovertible evidence. If you have such evidence, it is important that you report it.

There are other ways to be guilty of fraud. The most distressing case I know of involved a young, aggressive surgeon. He was highly recommended to us, and his record was impressive. When he was interviewed, he presented himself well, and everyone favored hiring him as quickly as possible because we really needed someone with his subspecialty expertise. After he had been there a short while, we were horrified. He went up and down the hall talking to the other surgeons, asking them to refer their patients to him for the slightest indications in his subspecialty. He then began to do surgery for minor indications and do more surgery than indicated so that he could charge more. It was difficult to accept that anyone would be so driven by greed that he would do the things this man did, but the evidence was overwhelming. Talking to him and trying to discourage this sort of thing was of no use, and he was ultimately fired.

Another aspect of following the rules involves honesty. My father always stressed the importance of honesty to me, and my worst punishments ensued when I was caught being dishonest. It did not take too many times to learn that lying is a stupid thing to do. In a later chapter, I will give you an example of how dishonesty can really hurt you, but for now, I would like to give you an example of a marvelous case of honesty. We had an OR janitor who worked evenings. He was mentally challenged, in that he was of marginal intelligence, but he was dependable, hardworking, trustworthy, and honest. One evening, while cleaning the operating rooms, he accidently tipped over an anesthesia machine. It takes a pretty good shove to do that because the machines are designed to be difficult to tip over, but a wheel evidently stuck, and the machine fell on its side when he gave it a push. He quickly turned the machine upright. Many other people, not wanting to get into trouble for doing something like this, would have said nothing. Fortunately for us, this man immediately sought out the nursing supervisor who, in turn, notified the anesthesiologist on call and told him what had happened. His doing this may have saved the life of the first person scheduled to be anesthetized with that machine the next morning. When an anesthesia machine of the sort we had is tipped over, full-strength anesthesia liquid can get into the delivery lines, bypassing the circuit meant to dilute them. Instead of breathing 2 to 4 percent anesthetic gas, the patient could have been breathing 20 to 30 percent, a concentration that would prove fatal after just a few breaths. The anesthesiologist on call came in and treated the machine properly to prevent that from happening, but if we had not known that the machine had tipped over, we would not have had a chance to correct it. The janitor's honesty and correct action in telling someone what he had done were crucial in preventing disaster. None of us scolded him for tipping the machine over, but we gave him plenty of thanks and pats on the back for reporting it to us right away. Honesty is always the best policy. If you make an error, stand up, admit it, learn from it, and move on. Lies do not prevent disasters, more often leading to them. The janitor may not have been brilliant, but he was honest. I will take honesty over brilliance any day.

Follow the rules. It does not cost anything to do so, and it prevents a lot of grief for you and for others. If you have a serious problem with rules that you have a chance to change, such as bylaws, change them if you can. It will take some work, but if you have a legitimate reason for the change, it will be worth the effort, because others, no doubt, feel as you do. It takes a long time to become a practicing physician, nurse, or other provider. It seems an incredible waste to end a career because of fraud, sexual deviancy, theft, and other unethical and illegal behaviors that are so unnecessary. Intelligent, educated, and previously ethical individuals sometimes end up doing things that no one would have suspected them capable of doing. Never get caught in that trap. Be honest in all your dealings, and do not overcharge. Charge for what you are entitled to receive and have good documentation to back it up. There is plenty of work to do to keep you out of the poorhouse. It is not worth it to break the rules and risk losing your job, losing your privileges, losing your license, being forced into bankruptcy, or going to jail.

Let's end on a lighter note. Here is a true story involving a notorious rule breaker. One of my fellow interns went to the admitting office one afternoon to pick up the list of patients being admitted to his service. It so happened that the local mob boss was being admitted at that very moment. This man was well known in the community because his name and face were regularly in the local media. In addition, he had a chronic heart condition that resulted in his frequently being a patient in our hospital. The intern heard this exchange:

Admitting clerk: And what is your occupation, sir?
Mob boss: Hey, lady! Don't ya read the newspapers? I'm a crook!

America is a paradise of lawyers.
—David Brewer

Make crime pay. Become a lawyer.
—Will Rogers

Chapter 9

Medical-Legal Issues

Elk and buffalo are constantly aware of the wolves hanging out at the periphery of the herd. You will soon become aware of the trial lawyers who earn their livings by suing the medical profession, constantly nipping at our heels and hanging over our heads like the proverbial sword of Damocles. Their professed goals are to keep us honest and prevent us from harming people, making sure that we pay through the nose if we stray. Some have even bragged egotistically that they alone are responsible for the improvements in medical care in the last fifty years, advances stemming from the fear of being sued. This chapter explores some of the medical-legal issues facing us. I will relate some of my own experiences, offer some ideas of how the system could be made better, and then explain why my thoughts will never see the light of day outside of this book. I will end with some good advice. While this chapter is addressed primarily to physicians, other providers should take heed, because you are almost as vulnerable as we are—the only real difference being that we have deeper pockets.

I need to say a few things about lawyers to begin. First, I respect them. My three children graduated from law school and passed the bar successfully on the first try, and I am extremely proud of them. Two of them are practicing attorneys: one a prosecutor for the city of Minneapolis and one a specialist in trusts and estate planning in a large firm in Minneapolis. The third uses his legal training daily in his business. We need attorneys for many things, and if you are ever sued, you will recognize just how much you need one. They are trained completely differently than we physicians. We are trained in the scientific method and in its specific application to the diagnosis and treatment of diseases. Lawyers who specialize in trial work are taught to be adversaries, to argue, and to win. Most doctors do not really like to fight and generally avoid doing so as much as possible. I will fight clinical challenges to the death but would much prefer to have my fellow physicians fighting with me rather than against me. Trial attorneys love to fight and are argumentative with a capital *A*. They are especially turned on when fighting each other, like bull moose in rut. In criminal cases, defense lawyers are taught that their job is to bring in a verdict of not guilty for the client, regardless of whether or not the client is actually guilty. They are further taught that justice is a product of the court system and that guilt is something determined by juries and judges, not lawyers. In spite of what I told you in the first paragraph, the true objective of the plaintiff's attorney in a tort proceeding, such as a malpractice trial, is to make money. Let me state it again as clearly as I can: The real goal of the plaintiff's representative in a lawsuit is to make money—to receive 33 to 40 percent of the recovery from a settlement or jury award. If you are ever sued or hired as an expert witness, you must remember that you are now involved in a game devised by lawyers for lawyers and controlled completely by them, a game whose sole purpose is money. You are merely a pawn in that game and should listen carefully to your attorney. To do otherwise is medical-legal suicide. Never underestimate an attorney. Quite often, they have as much book knowledge as you do about the medical aspects of the case, sometimes even more.

One rainy spring day, I came home from the hospital about suppertime, and Arline handed me a large envelope. She said that a process server had been there a short time before and left it for me. I sat down with a feeling of doom, and, with hands shaking as I opened the envelope, I pulled out a stack of papers and read the first page. It was a lawsuit. I read the list of defendants, and there was my name along with eleven of my colleagues. I could not imagine why twelve doctors were being named in one lawsuit. No wonder they call them shotgun suits, I thought to myself. Any physician whose name appeared in the patient's record apparently made it on the list. I read and reread the name of the plaintiff, but it took me a few seconds to remember who this individual was. When I did, I was even more shocked because I then remembered the case, which had occurred nearly two years earlier, and knew that I had done nothing wrong in caring for this patient. As I read the accusations outlined in the suit, I was flabbergasted. They had no connection with reality as I remembered the situation. Who made this stuff up anyway? Here are the facts of the case, and then I will explain how the suit turned out.

The patient was a woman in her mid-thirties who had been involved in an auto accident. She was rear-ended and got out of her car to examine the damage. When she did, she was hit by a second car and suffered a broken leg and some other injuries. As it turned out, the driver of the second car had been drinking at a local tavern, and the patient's husband successfully sued him and the bar owner under Iowa's dram shop law before turning his sights on us. The patient was taken to the hospital where she was examined and placed in a temporary cast. There was some concern about her abdomen, and the surgeon who examined her felt that she might have injuries to both liver and spleen. As she was stable without ongoing signs of internal bleeding, he elected to simply observe her. A couple of days later, when she was still stable, the orthopedic surgeon manipulated her fractured leg under general anesthesia and applied the definitive cast. A few days after the manipulation and casting, when the nurse was helping the patient to get on the commode in her room, she became quite diaphoretic and passed out. The nurse called the cardiac arrest code, and a number of people responded and helped get her into bed. The first internist to arrive recognized that she was not in cardiac arrest, but that she did appear quite ill. His immediate presumptive diagnosis was a pulmonary embolus, a blood clot to the lung. Quite a crowd had gathered at this point, including nurses, paramedics, and one of my anesthesia partners, and, out in the hallway, another internist appeared, who literally could not get into the room because so many people were in the way. He asked his colleague in the room if he needed any help and was told no, so he went away. One of the nurses dutifully noted in the record that he had been there. The patient was taken to the intensive care unit, placed on monitors, and given oxygen. My partner, who was on call that Friday night, asked me to come and see her with him because I was on call for the weekend.

Normally a person with a presumptive diagnosis of pulmonary embolus is given intravenous heparin, a drug to prevent further blood clot formation. The general surgeon and internist consulted and decided that heparin was not indicated in this instance due to her possible liver and spleen injuries and her fresh fracture, because heparin could initiate severe or even fatal bleeding under these circumstances. They also discussed taking her to the operating room to do an inferior vena cava interruption procedure to prevent any further clots from going from the legs to the lungs but decided it would be best to allow her to get past this initial episode a little more before taking that step.

On Saturday morning, I saw the patient, and she was doing pretty well. We measured her arterial blood gases to judge the ability of her lungs to oxygenate the blood and get rid of carbon dioxide, and all was well there. The surgeon and internist were still debating whether to heparinize her or take her to surgery, but it basically appeared as a damned-if-you-do-damned-if-you-don't situation. That afternoon, I was called to the hospital because she had suffered cardiac arrest. When I arrived, CPR was being performed, and all the accepted and appropriate treatments for cardiac arrest were given. In spite of those efforts, she did not respond and was pronounced dead. A postmortem examination demonstrated a large blood clot in the main arteries to the lungs, a so-called saddle embolus, as well as partially healed lacerations of the liver and spleen. The left ovarian vein was dilated and empty, presumably the source of the fatal clot, as there were no clots found in the femoral veins coming from the legs.

It is extremely difficult to describe the emotions that befall you when you get sued. Before those papers arrive, you feel that you are doing your best, working hard, loved by your family, and esteemed by colleagues, nurses, and patients. Suddenly, all that seems to vaporize when that document written in legalese comes to your door. Then the news of the lawsuit hits the front page of the local paper, and everyone in town who reads it thinks that you are guilty of malpractice, or at least in your mind they do. You feel nearly incapable of continuing to work, knowing that you are being sued even though you are confident deep in your soul that you did nothing wrong. You would like to say to your next patient, "I'll be happy to take care of you and do my very best, but please promise you won't sue me!" You want to scream to the world, "I didn't do it!" Your feeling of self-worth takes a radical nosedive, and depression begins to settle in with the force of a haymaker to the gut from George Foreman. Even looking people in the eye becomes awkward. It is no mystery to me that physicians have attempted suicide after being sued, sometimes successfully. If you survive the initial shock and depression caused by this monumental slap in the face, you come up in a fighting mood, ready to erase the blot on your escutcheon. It is then that you get a second slap: you are not in control. Instead, you have to put your faith in the attorney assigned to the case by the insurance company, someone you have never met and about whom you know nothing. Patients facing radical surgery, no doubt, feel the same about their anesthesiologists and surgeons about whom they know little. In a lawsuit, you become an unwilling participant in a battle between two opposing sides, one trying to get as much money from you as possible and the other trying to prevent that from happening, while your goals are to preserve your reputation and vindicate your actions; nonetheless, all you can do is follow the instructions of your attorney and let the game play out. How it ends will not depend so much on you, the merits of the case, or the quality of the expert witnesses, but instead on the argumentative skills of the lawyers involved and the reaction of twelve people to their arguments. It strikes you rather hard again when you realize that those twelve people know virtually nothing about the practice of medicine. The ultimate outcome will also depend on factors you may not even have imagined, as you shall see.

The insurance company assigned an attorney from Des Moines to our case. He impressed me from the moment we shook hands. He was a hardy, well-met, vigorous sort of fellow who inspired optimism and confidence from the beginning. He was an official for the Big Eight conference in his spare time, and for several years after meeting him, I saw him on TV many Saturday afternoons officiating football games. I liked him. He gathered the twelve of us together, explaining his dual role of representing the insurance company and us. He offered us the possibility of hiring our own lawyers but made it clear that he would be in charge. After meeting with him, I felt no need of another attorney, rightly or wrongly I do not know; in any case, I trusted him. We discussed the lawsuit and received a warning that we were to refrain from discussing it with anyone but ourselves. He passed out copies of the medical record, told us to review it carefully and make good notes, and advised us to start thinking about whom we might wish to have as expert witnesses for the case. He told us that we would be receiving a series of questions known as interrogatories from the plaintiff's attorney and advised us that he should be involved with each of us in answering those questions. Following that, he explained, we would each be individually deposed by the attorneys of both sides, something he would try to have done at our own facility to reduce the down time for each of us as much as possible. Having never been involved in anything remotely like this, I did not even know what a deposition was. The lawyer explained that a deposition is a session in which both plaintiff's and defendant's attorneys ask questions of the plaintiff, defendants, witnesses, or experts with a court recorder present taking down every word and later supplying transcripts to all parties. In essence, depositions are major league fishing expeditions for both sides in which ammunition for trial or settlement purposes is sought.

After he answered our questions, we departed to further contemplate our immediate futures. There was not a whole lot of laughter among us I can assure you.

Answering the interrogatories was a pain. Basically, this is also a fishing expedition in which the attorney is trying to get you to make statements that he can then trip you up on during depositions or during court testimony. "Dr. Fanning, in responding to Interrogatory #3, didn't you state that you had two heads?" The depositions themselves were something else. They were held for several days in the doctor's lounge of our clinic, which enabled us to continue working and to appear for questioning when called. As my schedule was a bit more fluid than those who saw patients in their offices, I was able to sit in on many of the depositions. The plaintiff's attorney was a nasty, humorless, disagreeable individual who could have played the role of the meanest SOB on earth in any movie ever produced. He had a Hitleresque moustache and a grinding voice that reminded you of a novice driver trying to shift from first to second gears in an old pick-up truck with four-on-the-floor transmission. I never saw him smile, but deposing defendants seemed to be his favorite pleasure in life, giving him his jollies as if he were the hooded torturer in a dungeon in Spain during the Inquisition. My deposition was two hours long, about average for the group. I was asked questions about my background, including training, certification, and experience in my specialty. Numerous questions were asked about the case, both within and out of my area of expertise. Only a few years earlier, I had sat for my oral examinations for certification by the American Board of Anesthesiology, and I can state categorically that the deposition was harder than that by a huge factor. The poor internist who had merely asked if he could be of help in a crisis situation was brutalized. He was deposed for over two hours and made to read ECGs, to interpret laboratory results, and to try and answer questions to which he could only reply, "She wasn't my patient, I never laid eyes on her, I never read her chart before this lawsuit, and I never examined her!" The lawyer was having none of it and kept him on the spit unnecessarily for as long as he could think up questions to ask, as if torturing him would produce answers he was not getting otherwise. This guy even strolled around the doctor's lounge and found a "throw-away" journal lying on a coffee table. He picked it up and started asking one of the defendants about an article in this nonpeer-reviewed publication that had been lying on that table, heaven only knows how long. He followed this by having the journal marked as an exhibit and placed it in the record of the deposition. The next day, you can be sure that the lounge was cleared of everything but furniture before he arrived on the scene. It was easy to dislike that shyster and I did, even though he was technically just doing his job. I did not feel so badly about my opinions of him when I learned that our attorney felt exactly the same. This was my only experience as a defendant in a lawsuit, but I have served as an expert witness and given depositions and court testimony in other cases. This was by far the worst experience I ever had, but none of the others were picnics either.

The deposition of the orthopedic surgeon was another story altogether. He was the same orthopedist that I told you about in the chapter on rules, the one who ordered a Jehovah's Witness to receive a unit of blood. Unfortunately for us, honesty was never his best policy. His deposition was nothing more than a giant collection of lies and was extremely painful to sit through. The man lied as easily as he breathed, but he was a lousy liar because he was so obvious in doing so. He took it upon himself to attempt to "out lawyer" the lawyer, and it was a disaster. It might even have offended that dreadful attorney a little bit to learn that there was another human being on this earth who was more despicable than himself, but I am sure that he also licked his chops while thinking of getting this guy in front of a jury.

You will hear this over and over, but you might as well hear it here first. There are four basic elements to a malpractice suit. The first is proving that there was a duty to treat. This is seldom a problem, but in this case, the internist who was not needed and did nothing at all could arguably have gotten off by showing that he had no duty to treat. The second element to be proved is that the duty to treat was breached; that is, the care given was inappropriate, not up to the "standard of care." To prove or disprove this element, both sides use expert witnesses, trying to establish just what the standard of care in the community would be in this or similar cases. The third element is showing that the breach in care resulted in an injury. It is usually fairly easy to establish that an injury occurred. The trick is to prove that the injury happened because of failure to adhere to the standard of care. The last element is proving that the injury resulted in a loss or in damages. If there are no damages, there is no case. In our case, the first and last elements were obvious. We did have a duty to treat and there were damages (the patient died). While there was an injury (a pulmonary embolus) that resulted in death, we maintained that the injury was not the result of improper care; thus, the crux of the case, as is most often the situation in these suits, was element two, standard of care. Did we neglect to do what we should have done under these circumstances? We argued, obviously, that we had followed the standard of care, and we had several good expert witnesses on our side who agreed with us.

As the date for the trial grew closer, we began to feel more confident. We were pleased that our experts agreed with our management. As it turned out, the plaintiff's argument of our failing to do a vena cava interruption or filtering procedure was completely negated by the autopsy findings. When you interrupt the vena cava to prevent migration of clots, you have to do it below the renal veins, because these veins are the only routes for blood to get back into the circulation from the kidneys, which have an extraordinarily high blood flow. The autopsy showed that the fatal clot had come from the left ovarian vein, not from the legs. The left ovarian vein empties into the left renal vein (the right ovarian vein empties into the vena cava just below the renal veins), so interrupting or filtering the vena cava would not have solved the problem.

Just when we were starting to feel good and were looking forward to vindication, our attorney called a meeting to which eleven of us were invited, everyone but the orthopedic surgeon. We expected this to be a pretrial meeting with last minute pointers. To our surprise, he opened the meeting by telling us that he had decided to settle the case out of court for $100,000 and that the insurance company had agreed. This was another terrible blow, one that we had not expected and could not understand, and the question on everybody's lips was *why*? The attorney explained that the judge assigned to the case was very strict and that he particularly disliked alcohol abuse, especially among professionals. It was well-known in the community that the orthopedic surgeon in this case had a drinking problem, as I mentioned in another chapter. He further explained that after hearing this surgeon's deposition, he was not going to take the risk of putting him in front of a jury and having him lie, something the surgeon did frequently and clearly, thereby setting the stage for the jury to believe none of us. This news hit us hard, and we all felt a tremendous letdown. It was not relief because we would not have to go into court; in fact, it was more like having your legs knocked out from under you. So our case was settled out of court because of one man—a man whose actions in the case itself had nothing to do with the tragic death of this poor woman. None of the rest of us had done anything wrong, yet here we were, paying this woman's husband a hundred grand, thirty or forty of which would end up in the pockets of that pettifogging lawyer. I was not angry with our attorney at all. He had done what he had to do and what the insurance company wanted him to do. I was angry at the situation and at the system, feeling that I had been let down and that my escutcheon would forever carry the blot. I have to say that my views of the justice system in general and of the tort system in particular have been significantly clouded by this unfortunate experience. I hope you now understand when I say the whole game is about money, nothing else. This all happened over thirty years ago, and I have neither seen, heard, nor read anything since to alter my opinion on that score.

I would add that this case occurred before the establishment of the National Practitioner Data Bank. If you settle a lawsuit or lose in a trial now, the information is sent to and stored in this Data Bank. I can only imagine how I would have felt to have acted completely correctly and yet be logged into the Data Bank as having settled a lawsuit out of court, an automatic admission of guilt in the eyes of many. It is bad enough to have had to describe this affair in detail every time I have given my curriculum vitae to anyone. Being sued is something you can never forget. My sole consolation is that I did nothing wrong.

Medical-legal issues as well as product liability and other cases in the tort system cost our society a great deal of money every year, and the price to some medical practitioners is truly obscene. Professional liability insurance for most practitioners ranges from a low of under $10,000 to about $50,000, although these figures vary considerably from state to state and are highest in the surgical specialties; remarkably, if you practice orthopedics, obstetrics, or neurosurgery, you will pay closer to $150,000-200,000 a year in some states, such as Florida. The reason for this is obvious, when you stop to think about it. In each of these three specialties, a good outcome cannot be assured, even with the best care; consequently, they represent the geese laying the golden eggs to plaintiffs' attorneys. If your fractured wrist does not look exactly like the other one when it heals a little bit out of kilter, what are you going to do? You cannot sue God or yourself for a lousy healing job, so just sue the orthopedic surgeon who took care of you. What the hell, he has insurance. If you get drunk, have an auto accident, and suffer severe brain damage, just sue the neurosurgeon who drained the blood from inside your head on an emergent basis and saved your life. I read of a successful obstetrician/gynecologist who suddenly quit doing obstetrics. One day, he examined a patient, made the diagnosis of pregnancy, and then invited her and her husband into his office for a discussion of her prenatal care. Before he could say a word, the couple looked him in the eye and said, "Doctor, we want you to guarantee us a perfect baby." He thought for a moment and realized that even God does not do that, leaving him no chance of making such a guarantee. He quit obstetrics on the spot.

A baseball player who bats three hundred (three hits out of ten tries) will command a multimillion-dollar contract. In medicine, however, the public and the legal system seem to have the idea that physicians can and must consistently bat a thousand and that when things do not turn out as well as expected, it has to mean that malpractice is involved. That is an unfortunate assumption, because for the most part it is simply not true. What is malpractice? Cutting off the wrong extremity, pinning the good hip instead of the fractured hip, and operating on the wrong patient are all clear examples of malpractice. Is it malpractice to stick your head in a door and ask if someone needs help and then turn away when told no? Is a child born with cerebral palsy necessarily the victim of medical malpractice? Absolutely not, but the fear of being sued for this is exactly why the C-section rate in this country is so high, even though the evidence shows that the excess number of C-sections performed really prevents nothing. When I first entered practice, the C-section rate was less than 10 percent. It is now closer to 30 percent, which is patently absurd when you stop to think about it. How can nature have decreed in the space of my lifetime that nearly one-third of the human race ought to be delivered surgically? I knew one obstetrician many years ago whose rate was closer to 35 percent, most of them performed for "social" indications (he did not want to miss a dinner engagement). He used to tell patients that the babies were cuter when born by C-section because they did not have to squeeze through the birth canal and thus their little heads were rounder. That, in my opinion, is malpractice. How about postoperative infections, are they always the result of malpractice? I would argue that they are rarely so. You would have to be a pretty stupid surgeon to want your patient to get an infection after surgery, and I have never known any that dumb. The surgeons I have worked with are absolute maniacs for sterile technique, and yet infections still occur.

Could it possibly be that factors like diabetes, rheumatoid arthritis, AIDS, advancing age, alcoholism and substance abuse, and chemotherapeutic agents used to treat cancer might be blamed for increasing the risks of infection instead of the actions of the surgeon and surgical team?

The system allows doctors to be sued for the most ridiculous of reasons. For example, an internist I once worked with and who was an excellent practitioner sent a patient needing a complex diagnostic procedure to a well-known and highly regarded specialist in Des Moines. The patient suffered a complication and sued the specialist. She also sued my colleague, evidently for having had the audacity to refer her to that specialist. It bothers me that a lawyer would be so money hungry as to file such a suit, especially as he would have been just as eager to file the suit if the internist had not sent the patient to a specialist, and she had suffered because of that. Because the real purpose of a suit is to get money, the more physicians you can name in a suit, the better. Doctors are usually well insured and thus have deep pockets, so the more of them you sue, the more likely you will be able to squeeze something out, either by a settlement or by a jury.

One of the most tragic problems with the tort system as applied to medicine is that the majority of the money ends up in the wrong pockets. For each dollar spent on professional liability insurance, more than fifty cents ends up in the pockets of lawyers, expert witnesses, the court system, and the insurance company. It is pretty hypocritical in my view for trial attorneys to tell us that the purpose of the system is to provide restitution for an injured patient when the patient comes out on the short end nearly every time, collectively receiving well less than 50 percent of the money we pay out for the expressed purpose of providing for their restoration. The majority of malpractice claims are settled out of court, just as ours was. Of those that go to trial, the jury finds in favor of the plaintiff less than 40 percent of the time, the only crumb of good news for physicians. Jury awards are much, much higher than settlement ones, which is why insurance companies have an incentive to settle a great deal of the time. The system is broken and needs radical change, but no one seems able to come up with a better system, and when they do, the trial lawyers immediately shoot them down because none of them want to kill the cash cow. If you will permit me, however, I will take my shot at proposing a better system, one that benefits the patient for a change and protects doctors from wrongful and unnecessary suits.

If a patient suffers an injury that is clearly connected with medical treatment, a court-appointed panel of experts should do an initial determination as to whether the injury was caused by inappropriate care. Once the panel of experts has determined whether a compensable injury has occurred, the case should go to court unless a settlement is agreed upon. The case will be presented in court to a judge and a six-member jury made up of three physicians and three laypeople. I would require all physicians to be available for this duty and exempt from other kinds of jury duty. The court would draw the physician members of the jury from the physicians practicing in the specific specialty involved and from the surrounding states, not the defendant's state. The lay members could be drawn from the local jury pool. The initial physician panel reviewing the case could be specialists from within state and their findings would be admitted in the court proceedings. Both sides would present their arguments to the jury just as they do now. If either side hires expert witnesses, they would be paid a standard hourly fee determined by the court; furthermore, expert witnesses should meet standard criteria, the most important of which being that the witness is qualified in the same specialty as the defendant. It is ridiculous to have an obstetrician judging the actions of an ophthalmologist, but that can and does happen at the moment. The judge and jury would then be given time to deliberate and, if necessary, to do as much research as required to come to a decision. Matters regarding ongoing costs of care, loss of compensation, pain and suffering, loss of consortium, and so forth would be presented during the trial phase just as they are now. I would cap losses for pain and suffering at no more than $500,000, and the criteria necessary to prove punitive damages would be strict and specifically spelled out by law, similar to what they are now. Monetary awards, if any, would be given over time as directed by the court rather than as a lump sum. The jury would also present its findings regarding the cause of the injury. If true malpractice is involved, the defendant might receive a judgment requiring retraining and/or monitoring of his or her practice for a given period. If willful or reckless injury occurred, there might be a judgment to deliver the findings to the state board of medical examiners for consideration for disciplinary action or to the court for criminal action. In other words, if the physician has done something truly egregious resulting in injury, it should not just be blown away by writing a check. In addition, if the court finds that the plaintiff's attorney has done something outlandish, such as suing someone for sticking his head in the door and leaving when not needed, he should receive a fine and be reported to the bar for possible disciplinary action.

How will all this affect costs? In the first place, insurance companies would jump at having structured settlements instead of lump sums. Secondly, the physicians on the original panel and on the jury would be paid at normal juror rates plus a per diem for housing and travel and be allowed to calculate their financial losses during this service and deduct them from both state and federal income taxes. Thirdly, paying the expert witnesses an hourly fee determined by the court would amount to a huge savings, as some experts charge horribly large fees to be witnesses. Fourthly, by insuring the presence on the jury of qualified physicians in the specialty involved, doctors will truly have a chance of being judged by their peers instead of a group of people with little or no medical training. Attorneys may argue that this would stack the jury in favor of the physician. I would argue quite the opposite, because I believe that physicians are not likely to uphold the actions of those who are truly guilty of malpractice. In addition, the presence of laypersons will prevent deliberations from being totally in favor of the defendant. I would also give the deciding vote to the judge in cases of a tie, requiring the judge to be present during the jury's deliberations. Finally, plaintiffs' attorneys would only be allowed to charge an hourly fee determined by the court, and the defendant's insurance company would pay that fee in the case of a judgment in favor of the plaintiff. If the judgment were in favor of the defendant, payment of the plaintiff's lawyer would have been agreed upon by both parties ahead of time. If the attorney feels strongly about the case, he should be willing to take it on a contingency basis. If not, he will ask for a retainer up front and full compensation when it is over if they lose. I predict that few, if any, lawyers would elect to take cases on a contingency basis under my proposed system, despite their praise of this aspect of the current system. I hope I am wrong.

Why do I think that this or a similar system is a good idea? It addresses several issues, the most important being to insure that the bulk of the money infused into the system goes to patients instead of lawyers, expert witnesses, insurance companies, and courts. It also reduces nuisance lawsuits, because the attorney will have to be pretty certain that he has a rock-solid case before writing a lawsuit. It would stop many out-of-court settlements and hopefully allow cases to be determined on the basis of merit alone and not a bunch of side issues. It will end the "I've hit the lotto!" tone of professional liability suits by putting a stop to lump-sum payments. It would insure that physicians who are truly guilty of malpractice receive some kind of judgment and punishment beyond writing a check, hopefully with the aim of retraining and rehabilitation. These benefits of the proposed system would correct the worst wrongs of the current system and reduce the amount of waste as well as reducing insurance premiums and hopefully the cost of medical care going forward. There are many other suggestions out there for improving the current system, some of which would certainly bring about improvements and have already done so in some states; however, I will tell you why the system I have proposed or any other meaningful change will never happen in our lifetimes. You probably have figured it out already.

There are two reasons why such reform will never occur, money and politics (two sides of the same old coin). Trial lawyers are not about to let their cash cow disappear, and they back up their insistence on its continued existence with sizable political contributions. In the two years from September 1, 2008, to August 31, 2010, the attorneys and law firms in this country contributed $76,569,831 to Congress, while physicians contributed $30,501,799. Not all those funds were directed to legislation dealing with professional liability, of course, but it gives you the correct idea that lawyers contribute to politicians more than doctors by a factor of greater than two. In addition to having a leg up on us in the contribution department, lawyers have another important advantage: they preach to the choir. In the 111th Congress, 225 members (168 in the House, 57 in the Senate) listed their occupations as lawyer. There were a handful of physicians, at most. I have always felt that allowing attorneys to hold legislative office is the most obvious example of conflict of interest in the world, but we accept it without protest. You can be certain that laws are written for the advantage of lawyers; therefore, it is highly unlikely that any meaningful changes in the tort system are going to occur in the foreseeable future. I will simply end this part of the discussion with two of my favorite quotes, the first from Will Rogers: "We have the best Congress money can buy." The second, a bit more biting, comes from Mark Twain: "There is no distinct American criminal class—except Congress."

Hypocrisy bothers me a great deal. Plaintiff's attorneys like to brag that they are champions for justice and are necessary because the medical profession refuses to police itself. A neurosurgeon in eastern Iowa was a major problem. He had operated on the wrong side of the head on more than one patient and had done more equally outrageous things in his practice. Several physicians had tried unsuccessfully to get him disciplined through the hospital's medical staff; finally, the anesthesiologists in town refused to anesthetize his patients, a brave and serious action by them. Predictably the surgeon sued the anesthesiologists for restraint of trade. I remember talking with these anesthesiologists at a meeting of our state society. The story, of course, had been splashed in big letters in newspapers across the state. They were extremely worried that they would lose the case, knowing that the law looks unkindly at issues involving restraint of trade; nonetheless, they stuck to their guns, because they did not want this man practicing in their city any longer. The attorney for the neurosurgeon was none other than one of the most successful plaintiff's attorneys in the state. You know the type, the kind who chronically and very publically complains that physicians never police themselves and therefore deserve to be sued to keep them honest. The anesthesiologists won the suit.

In another instance, an anesthesiologist from a small city in southeastern Iowa was brought before the Iowa Board of Medical examiners for several infractions, including lying on his licensure application and malpractice. He was responsible for three people, two children and a young mother, suffering permanent and severe brain damage. To have one such occurrence in a practice lifetime is a disaster for an anesthesiologist. To have three such cases is catastrophic. I was a member of the peer review committee in anesthesiology for the Board of Medical Examiners at the time and was chosen to give testimony against him at the hearing before the Board. His attorney was another highly successful plaintiff's attorney, one of the most noted in the state. You know the type, the kind who chronically and publically complains that physicians never police themselves and therefore deserve to be sued to keep them honest. The Board of Medical Examiners yanked the anesthesiologist's license to practice in Iowa.

And the point of these last two stories? In law school, they obviously do not teach their students that hypocrisy is a bad thing. That is why they can rail at us about not policing ourselves and then happily sue us when we try to do so. That is why Congress can make laws that affect you and me but exempt themselves from the same. Do not sit by mutely when lawyers complain about doctors. They have as many or more shortcomings as they claim we do. Before you go labeling me a complete dummy, you should know that I recognize and fully agree that even the guiltiest deserve a fair trial and good representation by an attorney of choice in our country. I simply find it supremely hypocritical for a plaintiff's attorney who proclaims something so loudly and persistently to accept a case in which his client is quite guilty of malpractice and to fight the system that is trying to do what the attorney preaches it never does (i.e., police itself). Do not bother to remind me that John Adams, a staunch American patriot, defended the Brits involved in the Boston massacre. That was an entirely different situation that we can debate sometime over coffee if you wish.

I have been pretty tough on the legal profession in this chapter, and it pains me to remind you that the medical profession is far from blameless in the medical-legal arena. In theory, if we all did our jobs properly and treated our patients well, there would be few, if any, lawsuits. The operative words there, of course, are "in theory." I just attended a meeting where I learned that only one in twenty-five cases of actual malpractice ever result in a claim. That is an astonishing and heartbreaking number when you think about it, given the huge number of claims that are filed. You may ask how this can possibly be true. You will recall that I told you that in proving malpractice, the plaintiff must be able to show that there was an injury which led to damages and that the injury was caused by the malpractice. If there is no injury resulting in damages, there is no suit. If the damages are not particularly large (less than $50,000, for example), the plaintiff will have a tough time finding a lawyer to take the case. Suppose for a moment that an anesthesiologist takes care of a patient scheduled for elective hand surgery under regional anesthesia (i.e., an arm block). If the anesthesiologist blocks the wrong arm, he is surely guilty of negligence. However, if he apologizes to the patient and cancels the surgery to prevent compounding the mistake, there will be no lawsuit if the block wears off normally and the patient suffers no ill effects. If, on the other hand, the patient suffers permanent nerve damage as a result of the block, there will likely be a lawsuit with considerable recovery. If the patient happens to be a major league pitcher and the injury occurred to his pitching arm, the award will likely be well beyond the normal insurance coverage. Health care providers are not always innocent of wrongdoing, and no matter how the laws regarding the tort system are altered, lawsuits will always be with us. Clinical medicine is far from an exact science, in addition to which, nature frequently throws us curve balls. People will always be upset with less than a perfect result, no matter how perfect and competent the care. Don't expect doctors to be immune from lawsuits any time soon. To avoid being sued or losing a suit, it is essential that you do your best to provide compassionate, competent, and appropriate care.

Enough. Let us end this dreary chapter with some constructive advice about medical-legal issues.

(1) Know your stuff. There is an old cliché that the best defense is a good offense. Defend yourself by knowing what you are doing and by keeping up with the latest knowledge and technology. Even if you are 100 percent in keeping this advice, you may still be sued; however, you will be well prepared to defend yourself. Take the time to do research in the area involved in the lawsuit. Make yourself become as formidable an expert on the subject as possible. This will help you advise your attorney if the plaintiff's expert says something off the wall.

(2) Be nice to your patients. We talked about this in an earlier chapter, but it bears repeating. Treat your patients with love and respect. Listen to them and be sure that you talk to them in terms they can understand and in language that demonstrates care and compassion. You want your patients to like you, not just to avoid a lawsuit but because it is the right thing to do; nevertheless, being nice to your patients does reduce the chance of being sued.

(3) Document, document, document. Another old adage in medicine: if it is not written down, it has not been done. It is pretty hard to defend yourself with the record if nothing is written in it. If there is an untoward event, such as an unexpected cardiac arrest or some other unanticipated catastrophe, take the time to write or dictate a detailed note describing exactly what happened and keep a copy for your own records. Never try to alter the record after the fact, unless you are particularly fond of committing legal suicide. A good attorney armed with a good record is a formidable combination in your defense. Make certain that your attorney is well armed. Remember also that most suits are not initiated until very near the end of the statute of limitations, most often two years in the case of adults, depending on the state in which you live. In two years, your memory of events will probably be like kimchee in a crock buried deeply underground; i.e., thoroughly pickled. A well-written, accurate, and complete record will help you recall exactly what happened. A good record will also be of enormous value to your expert witnesses. I have read some astoundingly bad records and advised attorneys that I could not defend the case based on the lack of proper documentation. Ignore those who advise that

you should not put too much in the record so that you can make it say anything you want later. That is absolutely ridiculous advice. Document, document, document.

(4) Trust your attorney. I have made it clear that you are a physician in a lawyer's game, and you must be prepared to play that game. You are a pawn that will be manipulated by both sides, so simply recognize that you are not in control and do your best to follow your attorney's advice. Getting angry does not help. Being depressed does not help either, and I think getting yourself into a fighting mood (minus the anger) helps to overcome the depression that naturally comes with being sued. You will not be accustomed to an adversarial environment. For your attorney, such an environment is like Br'er Rabbit in the briar patch—he is at home.

(5) Finally, remember that it is all about money. One side is going to try and make you look like an idiot while the other is going to make you sound like the second coming. Do not take it personally. You are just part of the scenery. The lawyers are fighting each other and will do about anything they can to achieve victory; that is, anything within the law, which is why there is a judge sitting there. Ultimately, the plaintiff's attorney is trying to rake in a whole bunch of cash, both for himself and his client, and yours is trying to save a whole bunch of money for the insurance company. If you are convinced that you have done nothing wrong, live with whatever happens. If you lose and you know you have done nothing wrong, chalk it up as being another victim of the system and be thankful you have paid your insurance premiums.

After all that, we need a joke. St. Peter and Satan had been arguing for centuries over the boundary between heaven and hell. It was a heated debate, one that particularly annoyed St. Peter. One day he had enough and finally screamed at the Devil: "That's it, Old Screw! I'm through arguing with you. I'm going to sue!" Satan turned to St. Peter with a wicked smile and replied, "Go ahead, Petey, old boy! Where you gonna get a lawyer?"

*Because I've been on the receiving end of infidelity,
I know how much it hurts.*

—Rachel Hunter

Chapter 10

Ignore Your Gonads

Because of your age on entering training, I know that the title of this chapter grabbed your attention; in fact, you may be reading it first in preference to any of the others. That's all right because I think it is a very important chapter, one that will no doubt stir up a bit of controversy, if anybody ever reads it. Hell, what's the fun of living if you can't be a little controversial? You will find, however, that I am not controversial in the avant-garde direction on the subject of sex—a subject that poets, songwriters, dramatists, and artists idealize and romanticize and upon which they insist freedom of expression and practice. I am not a modern freethinker with the credo "If it feels good, do it." My intention is to get into your DNA and tweak it a little bit to make you think with and be controlled by the wonderful organ shaped like a giant walnut lying between your ears instead of those little ovoid glands dangling between your legs or sitting against the walls of your pelvis. In appealing to your youthful procreative feelings, I would say that sex is obviously important, something meant to be enjoyed and practiced by two people in love; but in appealing to your rational, cerebral, contemplative, and moral feelings, I would say that sex in and of itself is not nearly as important as rational, cerebral, contemplative, and moral actions. Remember that I am preaching to you from the perspective of a seventy-year-old man who has seen a lot, much of it bad, when it comes to the subject of sex. I challenge you to keep this book and reread this chapter when you are seventy years old and see how much you identify with it then compared with now.

When I was an intern, I was on call, and it was very late at night. I was absolutely bushed and did not feel like going all the way across the street from the hospital to sleep in one of the call rooms assigned to us in the nursing dormitory. There were many rooms hidden in various parts of the hospital that contained beds and were available to interns and residents on a first-come-first-served basis. I came to one of the rooms that I had used previously and opened the door. To my surprise, two heads popped up from the single bed. The room was completely black except for the light shining into it from the hall behind me. I immediately recognized the two faces being bathed in the swath of light from the open door as belonging to one of the chief surgical residents and one of the OR nurses. I immediately said, "Excuse me," and shut the door behind me as I went to find another room in which to crash. The thing that troubled me was that the surgical resident was married and the nurse was single. Most people would say, "Forget it, Fanning, it's none of your business." It certainly was none of my business, and I have not mentioned it before now; nonetheless, I never felt the same about that surgeon again, even though I had highly regarded him prior to the incident. Because he was cheating on his wife, in my view, he was unreliable. I instantly considered him to be a liar and morally bankrupt. I considered then and do now that infidelity and promiscuity are virtually synonymous and are practices worthy of contempt. This view is not mine alone but is shared by the bulk of society, even by some of those who are promiscuous and/or unfaithful. You may disagree with my sentiments, but as long as you have already paid for this book, you might as well read on and learn my reasons for them.

If you are thinking that the example I just cited is a single, isolated incident, the truth is that there are undoubtedly millions of examples of marital infidelity. When Arline and I were having our premarital counseling with the minister who performed our marriage, he told us an interesting story. Because I was about to enter medical school, he wanted to alert me to some of the things I might experience as a doctor, especially if I became a family practitioner. It seems that he was called to a home one night in the wee hours to help intervene in a domestic dispute. When he arrived the police and the family doctor were already there. The story was that the man of the house awoke after several hours of sleep and heard noise emanating from the guest bedroom. He got up to investigate and caught his wife in flagrante delicto in the arms of a stranger. Now you might have thought that the brouhaha arose between the two gentlemen, but such was not the case. It was the wife who was causing all the fuss. She was madder than hell, but not just because she had been caught in the act. She was most angry because her husband woke up this time. He had never awakened during the past episodes she had enjoyed with her lover in the guest room. How dare he wake up and disturb them! This true story from the minister's personal experiences carried at least two messages: (1) promiscuity and infidelity are alive and well in America, and (2) traditional morality is not something that is universally taught, accepted, or practiced. You need to contemplate the consequences of sexual immorality if you are to become a health care practitioner.

As a health care provider, one of your prime directives is to prevent the spread of disease; therefore, you had better be firmly opposed to promiscuity simply because it is responsible for the spread of sexually transmitted disease (STD). It has continually dumbfounded me how this simple fact is swept under the rug in an attempt to hide its inevitable truth. Here's a shocker, something you will not see in the headlines very often, if ever: if human beings practiced life-long mutual monogamy, there would be no sexually transmitted diseases. You may take that rather long sentence and put it on a sweatshirt if you wish, because it is true. Mutual monogamy is demanded by the Judeo-Christian tradition but completely ignored by a huge percentage of those professing the faith; yet, from a public health perspective, it is the only certain way to stop the spread of STD. Anyone who approves the practice of promiscuity favors the spread of syphilis, gonorrhea, chlamydia, genital herpes, venereal warts, hepatitis B, hepatitis C, human papillomavirus (HPV: a cause of cancer of the cervix), human immunodeficiency virus (HIV: the causative agent of AIDS), and more. A famous basketball player who was infected with HIV once said something like this: "Just put that little cap on down there, and everything will be all right." He was referring, of course, to the use of condoms, and his implication was that wearing one makes promiscuity OK; however, his statement is like saying that a pair of water wings is as good as a cruise ship in the middle of an ocean. That little cap may be better than nothing, but it does not guarantee anything, and it certainly does not make promiscuity permissible.

In a bacteriological and virological sense, when you have sexual relations with someone, in essence, you are having intercourse with everyone with whom that person has had intercourse. Tragically, promiscuity is common, and millions of people worldwide practice it, leaping from bed to bed to dip into the cesspool of humanity. I hope you will not be one of them. This is hardly anything new, by the way. It has been going on for eons. Today, however, sex enjoys a tremendous amount of publicity, and we are surrounded with images and stories that make people believe that if-it-feels-good-do-it stuff. It is a terribly dangerous and unfortunate message on many levels. It is too bad that Hollywood does not depict its beautiful people coming down with STDs more often. You will never see a James Bond movie in which our hero walks into his physician's office and says, "Doctor, I have a strange looking painless pimple on my penis. What's up with that?" It may be chic to write scripts in which people suffer from AIDS, but the other realities of promiscuity and STD are simply ignored.

In our second year of medical school, we had a series of lectures from a public health specialist named Harry. I do not remember his last name, but our nickname for him was Garbage Pockets, because the pockets of his rumpled white coat were perpetually filled with papers, stethoscope, and anything else he could stuff in there. I had a friend who was a terrific artist, and he drew a marvelous cartoon of him, one I wish I had a copy of to this day. Harry gave some interesting lectures, but he was a bit of a drone, making it difficult to take notes from him. Fortunately, for all of us, a brilliant woman in the class ahead of us took superb notes and sold them to her classmates and to us. We all considered Mickie an angel because of it. This made it possible to concentrate much more on what Harry was saying and not worry about taking notes.

Harry's lecture on the public health aspects of sexually transmitted disease was a classic, based on real data reported by the public health official who investigated the case. He started by relating the story of several couples in a small town who decided to swap spouses. Everyone was disease free when they started, and it was agreed among them that no dalliances outside of the group would occur. This went on for some time, until someone in the group was diagnosed with syphilis. It was then discovered that other members of the group had syphilis as well. You will learn that for some people, especially women, primary syphilis is completely asymptomatic and may go entirely unnoticed. Untreated syphilis is a terrible disease that takes years to kill by causing disabling neurological and vascular disease. In men, the primary lesion, the pimple-like chancre, is often visible, but it is entirely painless and may be hidden beneath the foreskin. In women, it may be hidden inside the vagina instead of appearing on the vulva. Harry began to fill the blackboard with the initials of people in the community who came down with syphilis due to having intercourse with members of this group. These included a lot more than the butcher, the baker, and the candlestick maker and many more people than the members of the swap group, I assure you. Before he had finished, Harry filled a whole wall of blackboards with the first and last initials of people infected with syphilis resulting from the actions of one member of the spouse-swapping group. How did this happen, you ask? If someone's moral values allow him or her to spouse swap, what makes you think they would keep the agreement to refrain from straying outside of the group? Hell, if you cannot be faithful to your own spouse, what chance is there that you will be faithful to someone else's spouse?

The incident case turned out to be one of the members of the group who had gone out of town on a business trip. While there, he was invited to a party at a country club where he schmoozed a little too successfully and ended up bedding a woman he had just met. Of course, with his bloated ego, he assumed that she had succumbed to him because of his wonderful charm and ability to sweep women off their feet. It never occurred to him that she would happily bed anyone wearing trousers, as was determined by the public health investigation. He had taken that dip in the cesspool of humanity and unknowingly took the consequences home to his entire community.

This story is true, and the events did not take place in a subculture. This occurred in Middle America among educated and presumably intelligent folks (although not too smart, as it turned out). The story did not appear on the front page of any local, regional, or national newspaper, of course. In the first place, it would have been too scandalous, and in the second, it would have been an invasion of privacy. It is also probable that the publicity would not have prevented many people from taking that perilous plunge.

The public at large does not think much about sexually transmitted disease. They seem to have the attitude that it cannot happen to them. It can and does. When I was an intern, I was assigned to the medical (as opposed to surgical) emergency room for one month. One of the most common diseases I saw there was gonorrhea. It was almost as if we were running an STD clinic. Invariably, young men would come to the emergency room with the chief complaint: "I strained myself." On further questioning they admitted to having a discharge "down there." Physical examination confirmed the penile discharge and microscopic examination of a drop of the discharge confirmed the diagnosis of gonorrhea because you could actually see the gonorrheal bacteria inside of the white blood cells in the discharge.

Treatment of gonorrhea in those days was with a long-acting form of penicillin given as a shot every other day for five doses. It was important for them to get all five doses to eradicate the disease, because the discharge usually disappeared after the first or second injection. It was also important for the sexual partner to be treated. It turned out that I was the only intern ever to have 100 percent of the patients return for all their shots and bring their partners with them. The couples came in around noon to get their injections, and we began calling them the "Penicillin-For-Lunch Bunch." The nurses became curious as to how I was able to accomplish this. I did it through subterfuge. I told each patient that he had gonorrhea, also known as the clap, and that he would require five injections of antibiotic to cure it completely, and that his partner had to have the shots too. I explained (quite falsely) that failure to receive all five doses could result in his testicles and possibly even his penis falling off. No one questioned my warning, and every single one I encountered came in for all five treatments. I simply lied, something I am not prone to do now and was not prone to do then. Please do not lie to your patients, I beg you. In retrospect, I am not proud that I lied to achieve a desired result, although I ultimately helped each patient and his partner and undoubtedly benefitted society as a whole. Lying was the wrong thing to do, regardless of the beneficial results, but it was the only thing I could think of on short notice that might be effective. Today I would tell them that failure to adequately treat this disease might lead to serious heart disease, sterility, and even death. This would be absolutely true, but I really doubt that this warning would have had the same impact as telling a twenty-three-year-old that if he did not receive proper treatment he would lose his nuts.

I would be more than surprised if you did not encounter patients with sexually transmitted disease in your training and in your practice. It is a terribly real problem, both in America and globally, that regrettably causes an incredible amount of unnecessary suffering, sterility, and death. According to CDC estimates, there are about nineteen million new cases of STD each year in the United States with nearly half of those occurring in people fifteen to twenty-four years of age. This adds about $14.7 billion (with a *B*) to our nation's annual health care bill. I find it both tragic and ironic that promiscuity, a behavior that is considered unacceptable by most societal norms, is responsible for one of the leading causes of death and disease on this planet. On those grounds as well as on moral principles, I totally disagree with and detest anyone who champions the practice of promiscuity.

If you ask people on the street if it is OK to cheat on their spouses, they will probably say no, even if they are already doing so. Why is that? I think it is because monogamy has been the norm for so long in our society and because people know that cheating on one's spouse carries consequences. What troubles me is that even though many are aware of the consequences, they continue to cheat. Actually the roots of our sexual mores go all the way back to the Ten Commandments and undoubtedly beyond. The firm bedrock of the Anglo-American system of jurisprudence is the Ten Commandments (Exodus 20:2-17), and, even if you are not particularly religious, you probably know most of the tenets of that document. One of them is "Thou shalt not commit adultery." Now it doesn't say "It'd be nice if you didn't commit adultery," nor "Maybe you shouldn't commit adultery," nor "If you know what's good for you, you won't commit adultery." Instead, it says "Thou shalt *not* commit adultery." Whether you are religious or not, this is a rational and sound directive. In days past, before the loosening of the laws regarding divorce, the number one grounds for divorce in virtually every state was adultery, and in many states, it was the only grounds on which to sue for divorce. Adultery is still looked upon with contempt by most people, even the hypocrites (such as many of our politicians) who condemn it while doing it. As you have already read, I am certainly not fond of promiscuity, and I am just as disgusted by infidelity, even once.

In my opinion, after years of observation, I believe that marital infidelity is often a sign of weakness, animalism, egomania, and/or lack of moral fiber. I also recognize that some people have psychopathology that makes it quite difficult to resist sexual urges. While these are not the only reasons for infidelity, they certainly stand out above the rest. I reject those who say that infidelity is just a sign of a marriage already on the verge of breaking up and is therefore understandable and acceptable. I would respond to that by pointing out that an honest person of high moral character should recognize when a marriage is on the verge of breaking up and act accordingly. There are competent marriage counselors available to anyone who needs help if a relationship is worthy of salvage; but if counseling seems pointless, ending the marriage on as agreeable terms as possible may be the best solution. Adding infidelity to the mix is like throwing boiling oil on a wound or a bucket of gasoline on a house already in flames. It has no positive effects, only negative. If one is unable to resist sexual urges and is disposed to promiscuous behavior, psychiatric help is certainly available and appropriate.

Many things can be forgotten in a lifetime, but infidelity for the most part is not one of them. One transgression can stand in the way of happiness for the rest of your life and the lives of your spouse and children. One can recover remarkably from the loss of an extremity, but there is no recovery from the loss of trust. You would be wrong to think that I do not believe in forgiveness; in fact, forgiveness is an essential and central part of our religion, and in the Lord's Prayer, we pray, "And forgive us our trespasses, as we forgive those who trespass against us." Forgiveness is extremely important, because failing to forgive leads to hatred, and hatred too often leads to self-destruction. Forgetting is an entirely different matter, of course; and I stick to my statement that there is no recovery from the loss of trust, a loss that is forever remembered. Furthermore, there is no hiding infidelity. Sooner or later, the word gets out; and when it gets out, you might as well have published it on the cover of *Time* magazine. Of course, I must not forget the effects of today's technology. Someone armed with a cell phone camera can have a picture of you and your paramour enjoying an intimate cup of coffee at a romantic bistro sent to a social Web site to be beamed to the world in mere seconds. That picture cannot be destroyed and will be viewed by many of your patients as well as your spouse, who was home with your children when it was taken. Being unfaithful was never very high on my list of things to do, not only because I truly love my wife, but also because the look on her dear face when she read or heard of others' infidelities led me to know that if I were untrue, she would cheerfully put a slug between my baby blues. Others have done as much and worse. The name Lorena Bobbitt comes to mind, and if you do not remember that story, please put her name into Google.

Infidelity necessarily involves lying as well as cheating. Marriage itself implies mutual fidelity and faith in each other, even if you were married in a civil ceremony. Arline and I were married in a church with a beautiful traditional ceremony in which we pledged to each other, "And forsaking all others, be faithful unto her/him as long as ye both shall live." Now that is pretty heady stuff at age twenty-two, but I meant every word of it and do to this day when the "as long as ye both shall live" part is taking on even more meaning. Some people write their own marriage vows now. Have you ever heard one that says, "And we are each free to have intercourse with anyone we wish as long as we both shall live"? When people marry, society assumes that they have pledged mutual fidelity. That's what marriage is. If I were unfaithful, it would make me be a liar, because I would be breaking the marriage vows that I took freely in the presence of wife, family, friends, and God. I do not want to be a liar (despite what I just told you about my treating gonorrhea), but apparently, a lot of people do not find lying objectionable.

I was at a wedding reception once and sat at a table with two couples who were militant liberals. The subject of Bill Clinton and Monica Lewinski came up, and I expressed my disgust with his unacceptable behavior and his lying. In a scolding and harsh fashion, one of the women told me in no uncertain terms that it was none of my damn business or anybody else's, that it was something strictly between Bill and Hillary, and that anyone would lie under similar circumstances. Sometimes you have to cut your losses to prevent making a scene, so I said nothing more, knowing that this woman must be at least amoral and possibly immoral. Perhaps she was just blinded by liberalism in her defense of her president. What I wanted to say is that in the United States of America, the White House and the Oval Office belong to the people and that the president is merely a temporary occupant. I could have also pointed out that the people have the right to expect the president to act responsibly and morally—including telling the truth, and that a president conducting official business in the Oval Office while an intern is playing "Yankee Doodle Dandy" on his little Willy is not acting responsibly or morally.

Infidelity is lying. Don't be a liar. We have enough liars in Washington, our state houses, our city offices, sports fields, and Hollywood. If you want to be a liar and a cheat, be a politician, an actor, or a sports star. Society seems to give these people a pass on the usual moral standards, but it does not do the same for health care providers, especially physicians. We really do not need liars and cheats in our hospitals and clinics.

While I am optimistic enough to think that many marriages on the rocks can be saved by good counseling and mutual commitment to finding a solution, I am astute enough to know that in many instances, divorce is inevitable and even necessary for the good of all persons involved. There are many extremely valid, albeit sad, reasons for a marriage to break down, including physical and/or mental abuse, alcohol and/or substance abuse, compulsive gambling, child endangerment, criminal behavior, and irretrievably growing apart, to name but a few. When infidelity is the primary reason for divorce, as I have already said, the victims of it rarely forgive in any real sense and they never forget. What do you tell your kids? Kids, of course, usually suffer the most after a divorce, although sometimes the split means that the daily fighting between their parents stops, which can be beneficial. Some people forget that when you are married and have children, you are never able to separate completely because of your relationship to them and because of all the activities that necessarily involve both parents. It has always bothered me that a spouse who cheats does so for his or her own egotistical and/or animalistic reasons and completely forgets about the fall out on family, friends, and society as a whole. Divorce is costly to everyone, and infidelity is still a leading cause of it.

There is a more sinister aspect to sexual mores that needs to be addressed before leaving the subject: sexual abuse and harassment. All health care providers are honored by their patients with a trust that is given to few, if any, others. They allow us to examine them in the most intimate ways, trusting us to be strictly professional, completely discrete, and totally nonthreatening. Most of us, of course, take this responsibility extremely seriously and never think of our patients in any kind of sexual way. Not only is that ethically correct but also required by law. I am licensed in the state of Wisconsin, and they made it very clear at the outset that physicians are to have no romantic involvement with patients until two years have elapsed between the last time of treatment and the onset of the romantic relationship. Failure to abide by this will result in the loss of licensure. Physicians who are guilty of preying on their patients are dangerous, should be reported immediately, lose their licenses, and be liable to criminal action.

Here's a story hot off the presses as I write. An Illinois physician has been arrested and charged with soliciting sexual acts over the Internet in trade for prescription drugs. The man is married and has three children. Keep in mind that he has just been accused and not yet convicted and that everyone has a right to his or her day in court. If he is convicted of this heinous act, I predict that the politically correct, feel-good elements of our society will want him to get off lightly with a slap on the wrist and psychotherapy. I certainly agree with the psychotherapy. This poor man has a serious problem and needs skilled psychological help. Personally, I would like to see his license to practice medicine permanently revoked. He has violated a sacred oath, and I believe that the only appropriate punishment and solution is to remove him from clinical practice. Taking him away from the pressures of clinical practice may, in fact, facilitate his rehabilitation. If he is found guilty of actually having consummated a contract of drugs for sex, I think he should go to jail also, where he can still receive appropriate psychotherapy. If he were guilty of this kind of solicitation in his office with patients, then he should definitely go to jail in addition to losing his license. We have to be tough, perhaps even tougher than some might view as necessary, when dealing with physicians who are sexual predators. When one of us is convicted of this kind of behavior, guilt rains down on all of us. I want my patients to know without even thinking that they are safe from sexual harassment during my care. After a story such as this hits the papers, people start thinking and asking themselves: "How safe am I?" Once again this is what I meant when talking about the rotten apple spoiling the barrel.

Sometimes it is not patients who are the victims. Sexual harassment in the workplace can be a serious problem, especially if the unwanted advances come from a supervisor or other senior person. This kind of threat should not be tolerated by anyone, as it is often the mental equivalent of physical rape. An internist and I were once asked to investigate allegations that one of our colleagues was guilty of sexually harassing clinic employees by making inappropriate statements and gestures. As we were wrapping up our investigation, he suddenly retired and nothing ever came of it. It is not just physicians who may be guilty of sexually deviant behavior. A nurse manager in the hospital used to call members of her staff into her office, remove her shirt, and make sexually pointed remarks to them. Sufficient numbers of people finally complained, and she was discharged.

Sexually aberrant behaviors in the workplace, whether directed toward patients or staff, are completely unacceptable. It is important to be thoughtful and careful what you say and what you do. Many years ago, we told fairly lewd jokes in the OR sometimes. That practice has or should have stopped. A completely innocent touch, sometimes even a friendly pat on the back, can be misinterpreted and result in charges being brought against you without warning. I once gently tapped a nurse on the shoulder to get her attention quietly, and she reported to her supervisor that I had hit her. I was totally shocked. Fortunately, she retracted her assertion when confronted again by the supervisor. Overly risqué jokes and foul language are invitations to being charged with sexual abuse. I must admit to enjoying humor a great deal, and I am guilty of sharing all kinds of stories, some of which are slightly off-color, but far from lewd. I try hard to treat people at work with lots of love, lots of friendliness, lots of laughs, but no lewd jokes and certainly no sexual threats. You would be smart to do likewise.

I have to stop and digress long enough to tell you another true story. I was assigned to give anesthesia for a gynecologist who specialized in assisted fertility techniques. His first patient that day was a woman I had cared for once, who was returning for a second ovum retrieval procedure. As she was wheeled into the OR, she looked at me and said, "Oh, Dr. Fanning, I'm so glad it's you! I have a story for you!" Here is the story she told me, in front of the whole OR crew, of course. A couple met in the bar of a hotel. After a few drinks and lots of conversation, one thing led to another, and he invited her up to his room. Once in the room, one thing led to another, and after they had done their thing, she got up from the bed and went into the bathroom. After she washed her hands, she held her arms out stiffly in front of her body, bent at the elbows with hands and forearms pointed skyward as she went to the towel bar to dry off. When she came back into the room, he said, "If I didn't know better, I'd think you were a scrub nurse." She replied with surprise, "Well, I am a scrub nurse! How did you know?" "Because of the way you held your hands and arms when you went to the towel bar," he said. "No one but a scrub nurse would hold them like that." She nodded her head and said, "If I didn't know better, I'd think you were an anesthesiologist." With a look of amazement, he gasped, "Well, I am an anesthesiologist! How did you know?" With a big grin she replied, "Because I didn't feel a thing!" That is what I mean by an off-color but not really lewd story. The nurses I worked with thought it was a riot and did not let me forget it for some time. The gynecologist, a jolly fellow anyway, laughed harder and longer than I had ever seen him.

A discussion of sexual mores would not be complete without an examination of the tragedies of teen pregnancy and abortion. As a health care provider, these subjects will undoubtedly affect you at one time or another during your career; therefore, it would be good for us to look at these predicaments together now so that you will have thought about them when you inevitably face them in the future. To get an idea of the magnitude of the problem of teenage pregnancy, I recommend you read a publication by the Guttmacher Institute entitled "U.S. Teenage Pregnancies, Births and Abortions: National and State Trends by Race and Ethnicity." This can be found on the Web in its entirety, but I will cite a few statistics from that report here. In 2006, the pregnancy rate for girls fifteen to nineteen years of age (per 1000 population of that age) was 71.5, for a total of 742,990. In that same year, the birthrate for this age-group was 41.9 (total of 435,436). The difference is accounted for by induced abortions (19.3 per 1000, total 200,420) plus spontaneous abortions and stillbirths (10.3 per 1000, total 107,130). For girls aged fourteen and younger, the rate of pregnancy in 2006, was 7.1 per thousand, a total of 14,790. There were 6,396 births (rate of 3.1 per 1000), 6,460 induced abortions (rate of 3.1 per 1000), and 1,930 spontaneous abortions and stillbirths (rate of 0.9 per 1000). As there were over four million births in the United States in 2006, teenagers accounted for more than 10 percent of the total. Fortunately, the numbers of teen pregnancies have fallen in recent years, but experts are uncertain if this downward trend will continue.

Teenage pregnancy creates difficulties on so many levels. From a health care prospective, teenagers present with a higher incidence of serious pregnancy-related issues, including premature delivery and the hypertensive complications (preeclampsia and eclampsia) associated with pregnancy. A significant number suffer from STD and substance abuse. Many of these youngsters, seeking to hide their conditions, do not receive any prenatal care until late in the pregnancy, if at all. You may wonder how one can hide a pregnancy, but I have observed on many occasions women who presented with a chief complaint of belly pain who were actually in the early stages of labor. In each case, the possibility of the pregnancy was absolutely denied by the patient. A fourteen-year-old girl who becomes pregnant is considered in our society to have reached the age of majority, capable of making adult decisions and carrying adult responsibilities. It seems ludicrous that the mere presence of a gravid uterus automatically thrusts one into adulthood, but it does, at least legally. Suddenly, a child is faced with multiple serious decisions that she may be very ill equipped to make. This child may not be able to get her ears pierced commercially without her parents' permission, but now she is expected to decide whether to continue the pregnancy or seek to destroy her developing child with an abortion. If she chooses to continue the pregnancy, she must choose between keeping the baby and giving it up for adoption. She also has to decide whether to tell her parents or guardians right away or to hide her condition, hoping it will just go away. If all these things weren't bad enough, for many teenagers, pregnancy will mean the end of their education, making it doubtful that they or their children will ever rise to the level of happiness, independence, and success in life that they might otherwise have achieved. With all these facing a frightened, confused, and often desperate child, it is important that health care providers approach them with as much compassion, understanding, and support as possible.

It does not help to point fingers in too many directions to assess blame and guilt for teenage pregnancy. It is really the fault of society as a whole. In too many instances, our children are taught sex from a very early age. It begins in the supermarket basket as our babies look at the tabloids and magazines at the checkout counter. It grows from there to the television set, the movie theater, and the lyrics of the music coming through their earphones. We readily entice children to have sex by providing them with birth control methods and by giving them breast implants for birthday presents while laughing at anyone who seriously suggests that abstinence from premature sexual activity might be the best choice for a teenager. We let them wear bathing suits made of less material than found in the average man's handkerchief. We should teach our children about love, responsibility, fidelity, commitment, modesty, and monogamy. Instead we seem to teach them the glories of animalistic sex, over and over. As a result, we will always be dealing with teenage pregnancy.

In 1973, in the Roe v Wade decision, the Supreme Court made it possible for a woman to obtain an abortion legally in the United States. That decision has been a major bone of contention and political football since, and both disagreement with it and defense of it seem unlikely to abate any time soon. Again, as a health care provider, you will be faced at some point with the issue of abortion. I was in my early years of practice when Roe v Wade was decided. Practicing in a college town, it was inevitable that abortion would become an issue. I struggled for a while and decided that I was simply an agent and had no moral connection to the procedure. It was the patient who had made the decision and who would have to live with the consequences. It was merely my job to insure her safe management while she was in my care. I never really liked participating in abortions, and after a while, I began to like it less and less. The sound of the suction extracting this helpless being from the uterus and the sight of the blood and tissue in the bottle started to nauseate me. It must have had a similar effect on several of our obstetricians, because one by one, they quit doing the procedure. I stopped participating as well.

Some people will think me an unprincipled fence straddler for what I am going to say next, but I disagree with them. I do not think that abortion should be outlawed as it once was. If a woman decides to get an abortion, she will do so, even if it means putting herself into the hands of some unscrupulous character, who will do the procedure in a garage using a coat hanger. That is the way it was done before Roe v Wade, and it must not be allowed to happen again. Witnessing a young woman dying of uncontrolled septicemia after an abortion is not a pleasant experience. Let me emphasize what I just said, because I don't believe that it is stressed enough in any of the arguments I have heard on the subject of abortion. Some women will freely risk death to have an abortion, including putting themselves at the mercy of an illegal abortionist or even trying to accomplish the deed themselves. In too many such cases, death is the result—an excruciatingly painful, agonizing death. In spite of my abhorrence of laws prohibiting it, I do not like abortion and would not advise my daughters or granddaughters to have the procedure simply as a birth control method. I think that instead of teaching freedom of choice, we should be teaching sexual morality and the sanctity of life. This can be done in schools, churches, and homes. It would be nice if Hollywood and Madison Avenue would also demonstrate some morality in this area, but that is most unlikely to happen. What I do not want is for Congress to stick its nose into this most personal affair, because laws against abortion are quite simply sentences of death for many women. I also believe that it should always remain the choice of health care providers to participate in or to excuse themselves from this procedure. No one, because of his or her employment, should ever be forced to help in an abortion. You will have to decide for yourself what you will do. This is a difficult area, because the morality is not as black-and-white as the activists would have us believe. There are many solid reasons for abortions, including rape, incest, mental illness, and numerous other individual tragedies; therefore, I believe the decision should be on the shoulders of the individual and the person performing the abortion, not on our Congress. To many, these opinions make me both prolife and prochoice, reviled by both camps. I prefer to view myself as antiabortion and anti-Congress.

Learn to control the energy emanating from your gonads. Learn to control your ego as well. Do not be so naïve as to think you can get away with infidelity and promiscuity for very long. You cannot. Nobody makes it through this life alone. So have some respect for the ones who love, trust, and help you. You are obviously an intelligent person, or you would not have been admitted to study in a medical field. Use that intelligence to guide your behavior to control your most basic urges. You should act as a sentient being aware of right and wrong and not like an alley cat that knows no better than to act through instinct and animalistic craving. If you marry, marry for love and remain faithful to your spouse. It is the right thing to do; and you will both be happier and better off if you remain devoted, faithful, and mutually supportive partners in life. Your children will appreciate it too. If you are so unfortunate as to reach a point where divorce seems inevitable, do not let yourself fall into the trap of infidelity. It will only make things worse and will paint you with an indelible scar visible to family, friends, colleagues, and patients. It is an ugly scar and not one to be proud of. If you are not married, do not be promiscuous. If you have a serious loving relationship with someone that includes sex, please practice mutual monogamy, because the price of promiscuity—socially, psychologically, and medically—is not worth paying. Be smart, be faithful, be monogamous.

Do you now think of me as an intractable Puritan carrying a bucket of paint and a brush ready to apply the scarlet A? Considering the amount of disease, death, mental turmoil, and social upheaval caused by sexual immorality, perhaps a modest swing of the pendulum in the general direction of Puritanism would not be such a bad thing. Promiscuity is a hell of a lot more dangerous than secondhand smoke. You must understand, however, that the impetus for that swing of the pendulum should come from the talk at the dinner table, the Sunday school, the classroom, Madison Avenue, and Hollywood, not from the halls of Congress. Any change in our collective behaviors in the area of sexual attitudes should be a change in mores, not leges. I am quite pessimistic that this will ever happen, of course, because we have become a media-driven society, sitting as mindless as the Eloi, as we consume the harvests that Hollywood and Madison Avenue place before us. The producers in those modern versions of Sodom and Gomorrah are not about to change their offerings, for they have learned from and thrived on that most important of Freudian economic principles: sex sells.

I will end with a confession. There is something that Arline and I really have missed by being completely faithful to each other for all these years. We have missed a whole lot of grief!

*I still get wildly enthusiastic about little things.
I play in leaves. I skip down the street and run against the wind.*
—Leo F. Buscaglia

Chapter 11

There's More to Life than Medicine

You are entering a profession that will consume you if you allow it to do so. I have known many physicians and others who had little life outside of the hospital and clinic. It is certainly considered commendable when a person devotes his or her entire being to a profession, spending every waking moment grinding at the wheel. I find that kind of life tragic in some ways, even if the ones who lead such lives accomplish great things, which they often do. I do not mean to be critical of people who work hard—quite the opposite. The best physicians and nurses I know work exceptionally hard and frequently have to sacrifice personal activities to care for their patients. They are compulsive in their work and always stand ready to serve those who need their attention. I have encountered countless other health care professionals with that kind of dedication. Nonetheless, I look at life as a gift not to be squandered by toiling in a single direction if you can possibly avoid it. I highly recommend unhooking yourself from the plow and taking some time to enjoy the gift of life, and this chapter is devoted to examining how that can be done.

I am certainly not suggesting that you follow in lockstep what I have done; however, I do wish to emphasize that this world is filled with opportunities and amusements and that life itself is short. My mother had a little plaque hanging in her kitchen that I used to read every day. It was a picture of a little boy wearing a straw hat who had a fishing pole slung over his shoulder. He was standing outside of a window where a fresh pie was cooling on the ledge, and he was gazing wistfully at the pie. The caption of the picture read, "Through fear of taking risks in life, I've missed a lot of fun. The only things that I regret are the things I haven't done." Please don't reach the end of your life filled with regret. Take time to live.

We all differ in our abilities to concentrate and work uninterruptedly for long hours at a time. I recognized long ago that if I could not set aside even a short period of time each day to do something completely unrelated to medicine, I would go mad. It might be something as simple as reading the funnies, working a crossword puzzle, or having a pleasant conversation about sports, politics, or kids with a colleague in the doctor's lounge while waiting to do an emergency procedure after a long day of work. More often, when I was not on call, such diversions included conversations with my family, watching TV with our kids, attending their school and church activities, playing golf, or pursuing one of the many hobbies I became interested in over the years. All these activities have helped me maintain my sanity and made me a lot easier to live with, I'm sure.

I have indulged in several hobbies and diversions over the course of my life. I love photography, and, while I am no artist with a camera, I have taken many lovely pictures and recorded family and church events. I also became interested in astronomy and eventually ended up joining my love of photography with my love of astronomy. I have even had a couple of my pictures published in *Astronomy* magazine, something of which I am very proud. I also went through a model railroad phase, having not been the recipient of an electric train for Christmas in my childhood, despite multiple pleas and even begging. I am delighted that my two grandsons share this passion, and they race to the basement to play with the train when they come to visit. Finally, I have an enduring fascination with World War II and have read numerous publications about it and watched hours of movies and documentaries. Finding a hobby or hobbies is a wonderful thing to do, because it gives you new avenues for education, recreation, and relaxation. I highly recommend it.

Golf has been a passion in my life, off and on, for many years. I caddied at age ten or eleven and developed a love of the game. A neighbor gave me an old hickory-shafted five iron, and I used to hit balls on the schoolyard across from our home in Tulsa. I played a little in my teen years and in college I took golf as a carry-over sport in gym class. Through medical school and residency there was little time for golf, but in Iowa we joined the country club. I played a little while the kids were still in school, and only one of them, my daughter, Mary Ellen, took any real interest in the game. I still love to play with her and her husband, Steve, and my other son-in-law, Ted. When they were all in college, I began to play more often.

I was even blessed to receive that miracle called a hole-in-one on a bright Sunday morning—yes, after having gone to early church. I still love golf and try to play once or twice a week when I can. I enjoy it despite my total knee replacement and lumbar laminectomy surgery in recent years, and pushing the cart around the nine-hole course where I play is excellent exercise. There are many other sporting activities available for recreation, of course, and I heartily encourage you to participate in whichever one (or more) flips your switch.

My father never liked to travel. I cannot remember ever taking a trip with my parents in which we were simply tourists. Consequently, I was overjoyed when it finally became possible to travel and see things I had read and dreamed about in my youth. We took many vacations with our children in the summers. During the winter, we would plan where we wanted to go. I loved getting all the maps and making all the motel reservations. We traveled out west several times to places like the Tetons, Yellowstone, and Sun Valley. We took a wagon train trip in western Kansas the summer of the bicentennial 1976. We traveled with the children to Sweden twice and were fortunate to visit Arline's relatives there, relatives she discovered while pursuing her passion: genealogy. Arline and I have traveled to England several times since the children have grown and have been honored to visit her relatives in East Yorkshire. Traveling is a wonderful way to enrich your life, to see marvelous geological and manmade sites, to meet fascinating people, and to learn new things first hand.

Many humorous and exciting events happen when you travel, and memories are painted that never fade. I will give you one example just to make the point. On our second trip to Sweden, we stayed in Stockholm at the Sheraton Hotel. We drove up in our rental van, and an elegant doorman opened the van doors and helped us unload. He was the modern incarnation of a giant Viking, complete with a long red beard and dressed in a fancy uniform topped off with a tall fur hat. I parked in the hotel's underground garage. A few days later, when we were ready to check out, the kids and I took a load of luggage to the van. When I opened the sliding side door, the damn thing simply fell off! There were parts lying all over the floor of the garage. Talk about feeling helpless! I was instantly furious and let out a string of oaths that turned the air pretty blue. With a great deal of effort, I managed to get the door back on the van and lock it in place, but it could not be opened again until I had found some place to get it fixed. This meant that getting into the back seat of the van required crawling in from either the front seat or from the storage area by entering through the lift gate in back, as there was no side door on the driver's side. We went back to the room where two of the kids delighted in telling Mommy and Grandma that the van door was broken but that Daddy had "fixed" it. The third seemed more preoccupied with the new words she had learned from Daddy when the door fell off and wondered if they were some of the Swedish words we were supposed to be learning. The words were of Anglo-Saxon origin, of course, but bore little resemblance to any modern Swedish I ever encountered. The best was yet to come. We took the remaining luggage, and all of us went to the lobby. I drove the van around to the front of the hotel, and there was the elegant Viking waiting to help us. I screamed to warn him not to open the sliding door. The look on his face was really funny as he watched while my wife and kids scrambled into the car from different directions, including through the lift gate at the back. Grandma was physically unable to enter the van in such a fashion, so she and I sat in front. After throwing in the rest of the luggage and securing all the doors, we drove off. We laughed as we imagined the Viking doorman scratching his head and saying in perfect Swedish: "There goes another bunch of crazy Americans! Why didn't they just use the side door?"

You do not have to go abroad or take big trips to get your mind off medicine for a while. There are plenty of activities in the community that help fulfill that goal year round. Religious activities, school functions, service and fraternal organizations, sporting activities and events, and other entertainments all help to get you into the swim of life and away from the stresses of a difficult profession. You are intelligent and no doubt find joy in intellectual pursuits such as art, music, reading, writing, and all the other leisure activities that keep your synapses happy with pleasant mental exercise. Look around you, get to know your neighbors, and become involved in your community with friends and family. There are so many things close to home to enjoy and wonderful people to meet. There is a whole world of happy, healthy souls outside of the hospital and clinic. Get out and enjoy them! Your life will be much richer and you will be better able to relate to your patients like a real human being. Give your brain a break—*live*!

I know a man who gave up smoking, drinking, sex, and rich food. He was healthy right up to the day he killed himself.
—Johnny Carson

Chapter 12

Take Care of Yourself

In order to care for the sick, it is important that you stay healthy. While that may be easier said than done, there are many things you can do to improve your chances of being healthy over the length of your career. In this chapter, we will examine some of the more important ways to stay well to serve the suffering.

Good advice on staying healthy begins with this: avoid all tobacco products. As you start to take care of patients, you should be impressed with how many diseases are related to the use of tobacco. Every time I see young people smoking, I feel so sorry for them. The seeds they sow today will blossom into unspeakable suffering in thirty or forty years when it will be too late to do much to help except for intense measures, such as coronary bypass surgery, lung transplantation, and so forth. I feel equally sad for young people who use snuff or chewing tobacco. They should know that there is an unacceptably high incidence of oral cancer in people who begin this habit at a young age. When I mentally picture their faces after radical surgery, I want to scream and order them to spit it out.

When I started medical school, my father-in-law was just beginning his battle with chronic bronchitis and emphysema, a battle he lost about ten years later. My mother had already developed advanced peripheral vascular disease and was told by her physician to stop smoking or lose one or both legs. She did quit, but the ravages of the disease caused by her years of smoking ultimately took her life too. At the end of my first year of medical school, I looked at the cigarette between my second and third fingers and asked myself this question: "You're supposed to be smart. Who's in charge, you or that cigarette?" I quit that very moment, a few weeks before my final exams in biochemistry and physiology. Several months later, the first Surgeon General's Report on Smoking was published. It really understated the dangers of tobacco, and the list of conditions associated with the use of this noxious weed has grown significantly since that first warning. If you think smoking is a cool and harmless habit, you are sadly mistaken. Smoking is one of the worst addictions, one that many people are simply unable to conquer. I remember quite vividly the patient we found dead in the bathroom at the VA Hospital in Syracuse. He had gone into the bathroom to sneak a cigarette by smoking through the tracheostomy tube in his neck. It was a poignant sight to see him lying there with the cigarette still in his fingers, breathless through the hole in his neck and unseeing through his open yet lifeless eyes. Smoking is a one-way street to suffering and death. It is also an expensive habit and a very obnoxious one to nonsmokers. You will also find it difficult to be a smoker in the health care professions, because most hospitals and clinics are now smoke-free. Please do not use tobacco products. You will thank me for the advice when you see the devastating effects of tobacco use in your patients.

There is a lot of publicity about exercise and its health benefits, much of which is true. We are designed as mobile beasts, and inactivity is not good. My mother used to say that it is better to wear out than to rust out, and I think there is a good deal of wisdom in that statement. Medicine is a relatively sedentary profession, and even in our average ten- to fourteen-hour days, we fail to get nearly as much exercise as the average farmer, carpenter, or hunter-gatherer. Furthermore, we know that exercise is not only beneficial to the cardiorespiratory and musculoskeletal systems, but also to our psyches as a major stress reliever. It is difficult to work exercise into your daily schedule, but it is well worth the effort. You will not have to do horrendous exercises to stay healthy. Walking, bicycling, jogging, swimming, yard work, golfing (without a riding cart, of course), tennis, and many other pleasant pursuits provide plenty of exercise if done for thirty to sixty minutes at a time several days a week. That may actually be a tall order for a busy practitioner with a young active family, but it can be done.

You already know that I have never been much for heavy exercise for myself and have always disliked running, although I love to take walks and to play golf; nonetheless, I respect those who enjoy running and who are devoted enough to train for such competitions as a traditional marathon.

One of my former colleagues was into running and did so with religious fervor. One year, he ran in the Boston Marathon, a real thrill for him. As he was running, he passed a woman and noticed that there was blood streaming down her leg from under her running shorts. He said to her, "Ma'am, I can't help noticing that you are bleeding. I am a physician. Is there anything I can do for you?" She curtly replied, "Yeah, mind your own business!" I would say that she was a bit overly devoted to running, not an especially healthy situation. The marathon has rather fascinated me for a long time. Apparently, people choose to forget that the original marathon runner was a Greek soldier carrying a message to his king and that he dropped dead upon delivering the message. I have always thought there was a lesson to be learned from that; still, I cannot help but say "Hats off!" to those willing and able to train and participate in such events.

Exercise, like many other things in life, can be taken to the extreme. I once worked with a surgeon who was a triathlete. He was an excellent surgeon and very quick, but he got quicker when he became a triathlete; however, increasing the pace in surgery is not always the best thing to do. He would work like crazy to finish his cases in the morning so that he would have time to bike, swim, or run before seeing his patients in the clinic in the afternoon. It was obvious from his conversation that exercise was foremost in his mind all morning long, and I felt that sometimes he might be cutting corners a bit closely as a result. I cannot remember his ever hurting anybody in his haste, but the chances of doing so were always present because he was not concentrating on what he was doing as much as he should. Some people think that extreme exercise results in an outpouring of endogenous substances known as endorphins, compounds related pharmacologically to opioids. It is possible, therefore, to become addicted to these substances and to crave the activities that produce them (i.e., extreme exercise). The point is that in medicine you have to be absolutely dedicated to what you are doing when you practice and cannot let your mind and emotions be governed by a craving to be doing something else. Extreme athletes sometimes head down that dangerous path of longing for more and more exercise at the expense of all other activities. It would be wise to avoid letting that happen to you. It is good advice to exercise moderation in all things, including exercise.

We all know that overeating is bad for us and that obesity is commonplace in our country. I plead guilty of fitting tightly into both of those categories, and as a gastronomic sinner of the first order, I am hardly in a position to be preaching to anyone. On the other hand, I am outraged by the food Nazis, those self-righteous do-gooders who presume to tell us what we can and cannot eat. A low point came recently when a city council in California decided to ban Happy Meals at McDonald's fast-food restaurants. This is government gone mad, and those council members need to be voted out as quickly as possible, no matter how well intentioned they may be. The founders of our freedoms never meant for government to tell us what to eat. It is none of the government's damn business if I want to take my grandkids for a Happy Meal once in a while. I would never think of doing it on a daily or even weekly basis, but if I did it would not be the government's affair. Another example involves a school district in the Chicago area that decided to ban brown-bag lunches in favor of "healthier" cafeteria meals. I would not be opposed to their sending suggestions to parents for healthy brown-bag lunches, but to ban such lunches is an extreme abuse of government, an abuse I would characterize as tyranny. The members of that school board should be ousted as soon as possible. Over the course of my lifetime, there have been numerous food fads claiming to guarantee weight loss. There are advocates of eating only vegetables, no animal products. Others say we should eat only meat, "the caveman's diet." The truth of the matter is that we are omnivores, meaning that we have been given the gift of surviving on a huge variety of foods, a trait that has enabled us to live in an amazing range of environments on this earth while enjoying a vast selection of treats for the palate. The trick is to eat what you like and what agrees with you, eat modest amounts of it, and exercise appropriately. An internist once told me that runners do not really live longer; it just seems like it to them. When he took up running some time later, I asked him why. He said he was doing it so that he could eat more. I read this quote in an old physiology text years ago: "The longer the beltline, the shorter the lifeline." Be careful what you eat and get some exercise as often as you can, but I insist that you tell the food Nazis to go to hell.

Alcohol is a legal drug that has been used in Western society for centuries for both religious and social purposes. A sizable majority of people consumes alcohol at intervals varying from hourly to yearly. Its abuse is unfortunately quite common, and alcohol-related traffic accidents and deaths still occur far too frequently despite repeated warnings and more stringent laws. The problem is that some people are simply unable to control their alcohol intake, and once they begin drinking, all the warnings, laws, and dangers are forgotten. Another problem is that you cannot know if this is how you will react to alcohol consumption until you start drinking. If alcoholism is a common finding in your family, there is a pretty good chance you will be a problem drinker too. One arrest for driving under the influence ought to be enough to wake you up that you cannot handle alcohol. Be aware that alcohol is just as dangerous as any other drug that alters your ability to think and to act. The fact that it is available legally and that its use is socially acceptable makes it no less dangerous.

You cannot practice medicine for very long before learning the dangers of alcohol. I have seen few automobile accidents that did not involve alcohol at some level. One night, I was on emergency duty at the hospital, and two college students were brought in following a dramatic accident resulting from a high-speed chase with the police during which the student's car flew off the road and crashed. The passenger was thrown backward, breaking the rear window with his head, and was found by the police lying with his head hanging out the window. The driver's head went through the windshield, but he rebounded into the car. There were no airbags in those days, and neither victim was wearing a seatbelt. The passenger sustained a few minor scratches but was otherwise intact—a true miracle, considering that the police estimated that they were going about ninety miles per hour when they left the road. I have often wondered why he was not decapitated when he broke through the back window of the car. The driver had a very long and deep laceration on his forehead, and he was obnoxiously rude, foul-mouthed, and uncooperative. With a great deal of difficulty and with major support from nurses and paramedics, I managed to inject local anesthetic and achieve closure of his wound with many sutures, during which, he continued to swear profusely and fight us as much as he could, twisting his head and cursing me violently as I tried to put him back together as cosmetically as possible. It did not surprise me when the blood alcohol level came back over 0.200 (legal limit 0.080), but I was concerned that some of his behavior might be a sign of brain injury. I notified a neurologist and suggested that the patient be admitted for observation, and he agreed. When I was finished with the initial care, I called his parents who lived in a town some distance north of us. From the noise in the background it sounded like I had called a bar, and I learned that his parents were the proprietors of the bar. I explained the situation and said that he would be admitted to the hospital. They sounded grateful and said that they would be down to see him the next day.

In the morning, I went to his room to see him. His chart was in a little cubical just outside the door. His parents were already there, and as I reviewed the chart while standing outside of the room, I could hear their conversation. The patient was awake, sober, and suffering only from a major headache. The parents were telling him how disgusted people in their town were that the sheriff's department in their county conducted a raid and broke up a keg party sponsored by the high school seniors in a local park. Here was their son in a hospital bed after having nearly killed himself and a friend because of being four-plus drunk, and they were angry that local law enforcement officials were preventing high school students from drinking beer. Because I am a physician and pledged to be nonjudgmental, I could not tell them what I really wanted to tell them. If they were unable to see with their own eyes what drunkenness did to their son, nothing I could have said would have had any effect. Their refusal to recognize the disastrous results of alcohol abuse blinded them to the utter reality that their son had been millimeters away from death and so had his friend. They were also incapable of understanding that their attitudes toward the use of this drug had led directly to their son's predicament, which now included a major confrontation with law enforcement. I have seen many, many other examples of the tragedies resulting from alcohol. Suffice it to say that this is an incredibly dangerous drug, one whose dangers are far too often ignored in our society. Please do not ever drink and drive.

Never practice medicine while under the influence of alcohol or any other mind-altering drug for that matter. It takes all our brain matter working in perfect concert to do what we do if we are to act safely and effectively. It is no less important for us to be sober when we work than it is for an airline pilot. A surgeon is dangerous when soused, and an internist is a lousy diagnostician when smashed. Nurses, paramedics, and all other health care providers are no less impaired when trying to function while under the influence. There are a few good rules to follow when it comes to using alcohol:

(1) If you don't drink, don't start. This is especially good advice if there is alcoholism in your immediate family.
(2) If you do drink, don't drink to get drunk. Alcohol can certainly become addictive and continuously becoming inebriated increases your chances of addiction. In addition, it is childish, antisocial, and rather stupid when you think about it. Think of drunkenness as

soaking your brain in a big jar filled with alcohol or formaldehyde. Not a good idea.

(3) Don't drink and drive. Those four words constitute one of the most important public health messages ever written. You will learn the real wisdom of this advice early in your career. Please heed it.

(4) Never drink when you are on call or when you are working, not even a little bit. Some of the biggest challenges of your career are going to happen when you are on call. I want my health care providers to have clear heads and brains whose associative areas are not hindered by the presence of the short-chain hydrocarbon known as ethanol. Remember to treat patients as you would want to be treated. I hope that includes complete sobriety. We need to change the old saying about being as sober as a judge. I would not mind if my judge had a wee nip (one beer) with lunch, but I want my doctor completely sober. I hope you know I am joking. Nobody, judges or anyone else, should consume alcohol when they are working.

(5) If you, your loved ones, or coworkers think you are having a problem with alcohol, please do not wait for treatment. Seek help immediately. Few people can solve the problem alone, but proper treatment can work miracles. I have worked with former alcoholics who were excellent individuals, so I know it can be done. The longer you put off getting help, the less likely you are to conquer the problem.

That brings us to the illegal drugs. That phrase by itself ought to caution you against their use: *they are illegal.* Fooling around with illegal drugs will ultimately get you in trouble with the law and that may result in your losing your ability to practice. Some people think these drugs ought to be legalized. That is an opinion held by a number of well-meaning intellectuals; however, that opinion is of little importance, because at this time, our laws forbid use of these substances. I hope your education will allow you to agree that they should stay that way. You may think that it is harmless to smoke a joint. There are quite a few experts who would agree with you and a whole bunch who would disagree. Long-term use of marijuana is undoubtedly as unhealthy as long-term use of tobacco; nonetheless, the real issue is that marijuana is illegal. It is insane to get willingly into trouble with the law. The same warning, of course, goes for cocaine, heroin, and all those so-called designer drugs people find fashionable. When you learn of the unhealthy effects of using these drugs, you have to wonder why anyone would use them in the first place. For some people cocaine is addictive after the first use. LSD has resulted in multiple accidental deaths after its first use.

Alcohol is dangerous enough, but the overwhelming majority of people are able to control its effects by limiting their consumption; that is, by controlling the dose. With illegal drugs you consume a dose calculated by a crook! By the way, you should be smart enough to know that there is ultimately only one way to get illegal drugs: from criminals. Think about that for a moment. I get paid to give my patients the proper doses and to be there for them if something goes awry. The responses of human beings to drugs fit nicely into a bell-shaped curve, some people requiring more, some less to have the same effect. I have studied and observed for a lifetime to more precisely predict who needs less and who needs more, and I can still get it wrong. Not too long ago, I gave a healthy sixty-year-old man a dose of sedative that was not excessive by any means, a dose I frequently use in eighty-year-old people. The man stopped breathing. Had I not been there to initiate artificial respirations, he would have died. When criminals calculate the dose, you do not know how much you are getting nor will you have any idea what they have mixed with the drug. Some crooks cut their drugs with milk powder or quinine crystals, yet people willingly inject this stuff into their veins, often with fatal results. A pathologist from New York City once gave a presentation at an educational meeting at the University of Rochester when I was a resident. He had multiple slides showing people dead in doorways, in stairwells, on rooftops, and in alleys with the needles still in their arms, most of them dying due to reactions to the substances used to cut the drug. Other slides depicted the autopsy results of people who had died from the effects of infections of the cardiovascular system caused by the use of unsterile syringes, needles, and drugs. The sight of pus on the inside of the heart and aorta is not a pretty one. Criminals do not care. The crook is not going to be there to help you when you stop breathing or when you have an anaphylactic reaction to something he has put in the drug. Even if he were there, he would not know what to do or have any reason to help you while counting his money. You will not find any labels on his products that say, "The Surgeon General has determined that the use of crack cocaine (or heroin) is potentially injurious to your health" or "Sterility guaranteed." Criminals are under no obligation to sell you what they say they are and under no obligation to guarantee safety. They only care about money and avoiding arrest. Only a fool deals with crooks, especially those selling drugs that can and do have fatal consequences—frequently. Don't be a fool.

Talking about illegal drugs reminds me of the most impressive case of self-incrimination I have ever witnessed. We took care of a number of college athletes for a variety of injuries when I practiced in Iowa. One of the more common injuries was a fractured nose, frequently the result of a pick-up game or even an intercollegiate one. One day, a young college athlete came to the operating room for closed reduction of a nasal fracture incurred while playing basketball. He was large, muscular, and healthy. Our most common anesthetic method for managing these cases was to sedate the patient initially to a level of comfort and sleepiness. At this point, the surgeon would take cotton pledgets soaked in medicinal cocaine and pack both sides of the nose. Cocaine is a marvelous vasoconstrictor and greatly reduces the bleeding when the instrument is inserted into the nose to manipulate the fractured bone fragments. In addition, it is an excellent topical anesthetic. After the pledgets were inserted, we would place a mask over the patient's face and let him breathe pure oxygen for about three or four minutes, after which we would inject a sleep dose of sodium Pentothal® into the intravenous and then allow the surgeon to do the manipulation when the patient was asleep. In this case, I had sedated the patient to a point where he was quite drowsy and comfortable, barely responding to us if we asked him questions. The surgeon inserted the cocaine packs into his nose with almost no reaction from the patient. Just as I was about to place the mask on the patient's face to give him oxygen before putting him off to sleep, his eyes opened widely, a big smile appeared on his face, and he proclaimed loudly and with emphasis on each word: "Man! That's just like cocaine!" The room filled with laughter as I gave him the oxygen and then put him off to sleep.

Society gives us special obligations and privileges to prescribe controlled substances and expects us to respect them; unfortunately, some health care providers ignore these obligations and privileges by diverting drugs to their own use. The medical profession, the government, and the legal profession have determined that certain substances are dangerous, that their uses should be restricted, and that careful records of their use should be kept. Opioids and sedatives fall into this category, primarily because of the risk of addiction, but also because of the risk of death from their abuse. Diverting controlled substances to one's own use is unethical, illegal, and, in my opinion, immoral. I am not going to write a primer on how easy it is to obtain and abuse controlled substances if you are a health care professional. Suffice it to say that it does not take a genius. Abusing these drugs is as dangerous and unwise as it is to obtain and abuse illegal drugs. Recovery from addiction is problematic, and the recidivism rate is very high. If a health care provider can be successfully treated for addiction, about the only ways to prevent recurrence are to restrict the license so that these drugs cannot be prescribed and to retrain the individual into an area of medicine that does not have direct access to these drugs. I disagree with the kinder members of my profession in dealing with this problem. These people view this as a disease. I agree that the state of being addicted is a disease; however, it was not a disease when the practitioner took the first step of stealing and using the drug. That was an act of will of someone making a very bad choice and ignoring the rules of the system—rules that were spelled out carefully to us from the beginning and enacted to prevent our making bad choices in the first place. If that bad choice was the result of a fundamental, underlying psychological problem, all the more reason for that individual to be removed as a health care provider, in my opinion. It is immoral for a health care professional to steal and abuse controlled substances, and I will opine again that these individuals should immediately lose their licenses and be denied reentry into the health care professions as practitioners. There are positions in teaching, research, and administration that might be appropriate for these people, but not practice. Such treatment would not only be in the best interest of the individual (you wouldn't put an alcoholic into a job as a bartender) but would also send the message to all others that such behavior will not be tolerated. It would also protect patients from being treated by people under the influence of these drugs. Mine is a decidedly minority opinion in a profession dedicated to healing, and many would scoff at my interjecting morality into what they consider to be strictly a disease issue. I heartily disagree and staunchly stand behind my view. There are legitimate reasons for health care providers to require the use of opioids and sedatives, but in every case, they should be prescribed openly by a treating physician and used only as long as necessary. There are no circumstances in which purloining controlled substances and self-treating are permitted. If you are having pain and require an opioid, see your doctor.

That brings us to the next topic. If you get sick, go to the doctor. I am as guilty, as most physicians, in treating myself for simple things in which the diagnosis seems obvious, but this really is not a great idea. I write prescriptions for myself, but usually on the advice of my physician, and I never write for opioids or sedatives. You will get sick sometime during your career. It may only be a strep throat, tennis elbow, or a bad case of gastroenteritis. See your physician, because if you toss off a sore throat as a virus, sure as anything it will have been strep, an infectious disease you can pass on to your patients. In addition, the consequences of not treating strep are considerable, as I mentioned in an earlier chapter. As you age, the chances increase that you will contract chronic illness. Hypertension, diabetes, coronary artery disease, arthritis, and various cancers (including breast, lung, colon, and others) all happen to members of the medical profession just as frequently as they afflict our patients. Many of them are more dependent on the set of genes you have inherited than on how well you have kept yourself in shape. You will remind your friends, family, and patients that early diagnosis is important in reducing the morbidity and mortality of these conditions, good advice that you should heed also. It is easy to ignore symptoms as you work, especially subtle ones. I had a prostatectomy for benign prostatic hypertrophy a few years ago. I was shocked by the estimated size of the gland, and after surgery, I was amazed by the tremendous improvement I experienced. I had minimized my symptoms, a dumb thing to do. So let me say it again: if you get sick, go to the doctor.

I hope you stay well. Eat, drink (if at all), and exercise in moderation. Be mindful of preventative health maintenance, including vaccinations, colonoscopies, mammography, and so forth. If you have a chronic condition, follow your physician's directions and take your prescriptions as ordered. I have reached that glorious age where I am a consumer of health care as much or more than I am a provider. I truly recognize the wisdom of that old saying we so often hear around Christmastime: "It is better to give than to receive!" I want you to stay well so that you can take care of my fellow patients and me.

There are admirable potentialities in every human being. Believe in your strength and your youth. Learn to repeat endlessly to yourself, "It all depends on me."
—Andre Gide

Whatsoever a man soweth, that shall he also reap.
—Galatians 6:7

Chapter 13

Final Thoughts

I have poured quite a bit on you in these few chapters. Hope you didn't drown. I thought I ought to finish up with a few comments about some of the more important points I have covered, just to bring everything together.

First of all, as one dedicated to serving the sick, you belong to one of the most important and noble professions of humankind. It is also one of the most difficult. Not only is there a lot to learn and to keep learning throughout your life but, as I have repeatedly mentioned, you also have to do things that few human beings have the stomach to do. As you work longer in the various medical fields and observe more and more, you will begin to think of the miraculous things we do as ordinary and even mundane; however, there is nothing ordinary or mundane about injecting medicines into human beings and keeping them in limbo between full consciousness and death so that complex procedures can be done without pain. Opening the skull of a living human being, operating on the beating heart, restoring vision or hearing, repairing a badly fractured bone, replacing a major joint, making images of the insides of the human body, curing a dangerous infection with antibiotics, and thousands of other surgical, diagnostic, and therapeutic procedures that you will perform, witness, and/or participate in during your career—none of these are ordinary or mundane. Ours is a profession of miracles. If you do not believe me, get out the history books and learn of the suffering of our species before vaccination, antibiotics, anesthetics, modern surgery, modern therapeutic agents, and modern diagnostic methods. Welcome to the ranks of miracle workers. Study hard, work hard, and be proud to serve your fellow humans.

Expect good things of yourself and your fellow health care professionals. Society gives us a great deal of esteem, and we must continually conduct ourselves so that we deserve it. Few things disgust me as much as a health care provider who behaves in a sordid fashion. If you want the high regard of your patients and colleagues, you must earn it. If you set your goals as high as possible, your resulting good behavior and good works will surely follow. No one can live completely free of error, and no one expects that of you; however, it is truly important to make good choices. People who continually make the wrong choices usually end up making tragic mistakes with equally tragic consequences, both to themselves and others. We see stories on TV and read them in the newspapers all the time about people who make bad choices and end up in trouble. It is an excellent goal to avoid being the subject of a newspaper article or an item on the TV news unless the reason for coverage involves charitable works, sporting events, or a letter to the editor.

A recent event that was all over the news will illustrate my point. Teachers called in sick in Wisconsin and went to the state capitol in protest of proposed legislation that would affect them. Calling in sick when healthy is against their contracts, as it is in most occupations, so they were told that they would need excuses from their doctors or lose pay for the days taken. Several doctors appeared at the protest to write excuses for the teachers. Every one of us has a right to protest, including physicians. We also have a duty and a responsibility to act ethically and legally. Writing excuses for healthy protesters is fraud. Electing to be a party to fraud is a bad choice, an immoral and illegal one. Those doctors are simply liars and have brought shame on our whole profession, in my view.

Try hard to insure that your bad choices do not result in actions that are immoral, unethical, illegal, or harmful to a patient. If you make a bad choice, let it happen after you have weighed all the options carefully when confronted with a difficult situation and picked the wrong option by chance. Honest mistakes are a lot easier to live with than stupid ones. I recommended in the first chapter that you must learn from your mistakes and the mistakes of others and try not to repeat them. We have been given excellent memories, undoubtedly the best in the animal world. It is a shame not to use them. Be remembered for your good works, your proper behavior, and your loving attitude. No one wants to be remembered for continually making the wrong choices or for being guilty of unfriendly, unkind, or unprofessional behavior.

People in the profession of medicine who are constantly on the move frequently have problems, often of their own making. When reviewing an application for a position, I have been skeptical of someone who has been in six, seven, or more other practices over a period of a few years. That sort of frequent change is often an indication of a person who cannot get along with his or her coworkers, who has something to hide, or who is basically unhappy with his or her choice of profession. This is not universally true, of course; for example, people in academics tend to move a little more to climb the leadership ladder and moving for them often means a significant promotion. It does not include those in the military, either. Having said all that, I advise you to be unafraid of shifting gears in the middle of your career. I worked with an obstetrician who became bored after years of practice until he became interested in assisted fertility work and completely changed his attitude. His level of enthusiasm and job satisfaction skyrocketed. It was an excellent choice for him and a real benefit for the community. The cook in our fraternity house in college once said, "A change is as good as a rest!" Sometimes it is.

I switched plows at age fifty-one, not because I was bored with anesthesiology but because I was becoming increasingly distressed with my situation. I was taking extra call to earn more money to cover my kids' tuitions and to help a colleague who wished to take less call. Over time, the extra burden became too much to bear, and I found anger growing within me. Every time I was called in at 2:00 a.m. for a C-section, I was enraged. As I drove the two miles to the hospital, smoke was coming out of my ears, yet I had to stifle the anger before I confronted the nurses and, more importantly, the patient. I recognized that this was my own problem, not something I could blame on anyone else; however, it began to consume me. When I made the decision to go to another practice, the sense of relief was enormous; nonetheless, it was a bit daunting to go from a multispecialty group with several extremely competent and congenial colleagues in anesthesiology to a group devoted solely to ophthalmology where there was only one nurse anesthetist and me. While I missed my colleagues in Iowa, the change was wonderful in many ways because it allowed me to learn new things, to meet new people, to live in a new environment, and to have opportunities that I had never imagined. I also enjoyed the interaction with my patients with whom I could talk and joke while making them numb instead of simply pushing in a dose of Pentothal to put them to sleep. Trust yourself and your feelings, and if new opportunities come your way, be brave enough to explore them. Sometimes the knock on the door comes only once. Don't be afraid to open it. The wonderful fresh air you let in might surprise you.

Learn to be grateful. When you deal with people who have to fight for life every day or who have to live with severe handicaps, you grow to be thankful for life, for good health, for work, for freedom, and for the skills you have to help those in need. It is too easy to take life for granted and to complain and grumble over little things. I know that is true, because I am as guilty of doing it as anyone else. I was at a meeting in Bristol, England, where one of the speakers was an anesthesiologist from Archangel, Russia, near the Arctic Circle. He was astonished to see so many stone and brick buildings, because virtually every building where he lived was made of logs or wooden boards. He was also impressed by the room rates of the hotel in Bristol because the fee for one night was more money than he earned in a month in Russia. It reminded me of the old saying "I was sad that I had no shoes until I met a man who had no feet." It must have been a bit depressing for him to return home after all he had seen and heard in England. If things get tough or you begin to feel oppressed by the stresses of life, imagine yourself flat on your back in traction with your jaws wired shut. That kind of perspective will help you weather the rough spots we all experience.

We are so fortunate to have the many things we have in this country to serve the sick. Our hospitals and clinics are absolutely immaculate, even luxurious, compared with the rest of the world, including Europe. That will change under government medicine, because there will not be funds to continually upgrade the infrastructure, something that is painfully obvious in other countries. Happily we are starting out at a high level. Take a little time each day to look around you, note the beauty of nature, be thankful for the marvelous equipment you have available, enjoy your clean and pleasant surroundings, embrace your talented and dedicated colleagues, and humbly accept your own health and well-being. When you have done so, close your eyes, bow your head, and give thanks for all your blessings.

There was a song in the Monty Python movie, *The Life of Brian*, entitled "Always Look on the Bright Side of Life." The song was played at the end of the movie when Brian was being crucified and gave comic relief in a mocking way to the horrific events that were happening. The title of this song remains as excellent advice in this world. You are going to see a lot of very sad things in a medical career and it is easy to let that cloud your view of reality. When you always deal with the sick, it is natural to assume that the whole world is sick. Don't let that happen. That is why I wrote the chapter called "There's More to Life than Medicine." Get out among healthy people and never forget that living should include being happy, healthy, productive, and loving. Take a lesson from those you meet who carry terrible burdens yet remain cheery and optimistic. I once worked with an operating room aide who suffered from familial neurofibromatosis, a dreadful condition that had horribly disfigured her face; despite this, she was cheerful, friendly, positive, and hard working. She was also a heck of a bowler. I have worked with people who suffered in unspeakably difficult domestic situations but who did not allow their problems to affect their work and who remained upbeat and optimistic, giving the best of themselves for the benefit of their patients. It is so important to exhibit optimism, because pessimism is unhealthy and destructive. If you lose your positive outlook, you will lose your own hope and the ability to give hope to others. A health care provider must be a purveyor of hope and not a hanger of crepe. Hope comes with a smile, a warm touch, a kind word, and competent, compassionate care. Be sure that you never lose your capacity to deliver it, no matter how desperate the situation may seem. I once knew a pulmonologist from Turkey. This kind and friendly man had seen a lot of pulmonary disease in his lifetime. Whenever we reviewed chest X-rays with him that showed unusual lung lesions, he would say, "Could be TB. There's always room for TB!" I feel that way about hope: there's always room for hope.

In an earlier chapter, I said that a physician should be a teacher and that patients should be the most important students. The reverse is also true. I once helped in the care of a woman with rheumatoid arthritis that had rendered her virtually helpless. I anesthetized her for more than one of her joint replacements and came to know her well. She had terrible veins, so venous access for fluids and medications was a frequent problem. Anesthesiologists are used to being asked to help in such cases. Her disease left her susceptible to infections, and she ultimately developed infections in all her knee and hip replacements, requiring more surgery to remove the four infected prostheses. This was a terrible blow to her, of course, because it left her bedridden. It was also a blow to us because our institution had a sterling record with regard to postoperative infections in total joint replacement procedures. Following removal of the devices, she required long-term intravenous antibiotic therapy, a real problem for someone with delicate veins. Her orthopedist, one of my favorite surgeons, asked me to insert a central venous line so that she could receive the treatments more easily. You know you've had too much surgery when you are on familiar and friendly terms with your anesthesiologist. This patient and I had been through a lot together, and she always greeted me in the warmest fashion. On this day, as I worked to insert the central venous line, she smiled as usual and began to talk to me. Her comments went something like this: "You know, Dr. Fanning, when I dream, I am never crippled up with this darn arthritis. I always see myself doing the laundry, cooking supper, or playing with my children. Isn't that nice?" These simple words from this delightful frail little lady spoke volumes to me about the human spirit. Here she was in a situation that would have left most of us beyond despair, and she was able to extract something positive. In Latin class in high school, I learned an old Roman saying "Dum spiro, spero." It means "While I breathe, I hope." I know you will care for similar patients and learn similar lessons. Pain and suffering are part of the human condition. So is hope—a more important part.

Now that you have read the book, perhaps you have discerned the values that I hold most dear. The qualities that best exemplify them are honesty, fidelity, obedience, humility, devotion to duty, dependability, and altruism. Altruism actually combines most of those qualities, but it is difficult to be an altruist in the current age. The altruist always puts the needs of others ahead of self, but this is an unnatural act, because we are genetically wired to fend for ourselves and to protect our own existence. The only common exceptions are the selflessness of parents in preserving their young and the self-sacrifice of police officers, firefighters, military personnel, and other professionals who daily put their lives in peril for the sakes of others. Unfortunately, some parents are not so selfless, and the destruction of the young by their own parents occurs too often.

I said that it is difficult to be an altruist. This is because our society has over emphasized the importance of self, as evidenced by the practices of schools to pass children to avoid damaging their psyches instead of demanding that they perform to appropriate standards before moving forward. In addition, we continue to pour our adulation on sports stars, movie stars, and politicians who violate the most basic standards of decency, giving them status, attention, and riches that they do not deserve, massively inflating their already ample egos. Conversely, police, firefighters, and members of the military are compensated and appreciated far below those in our society who are worshipped and adored, but who may be evil, self-seeking, and immoral. When I was a youngster, our parents and teachers taught us that we are judged by how we treat others and by how others respect us. Self-esteem may be important, but respect for others is equally important. Arline told our children that we will always love them and that we want them to behave so that others will love them as well. There is no doubt that you will be judged not only by how much you love your patients, but also by how much you are loved by them in return. If you are not basically altruistic by nature, you will not achieve true excellence as a health care provider. Your devotion must be to your patients and to medicine itself, not to your own selfish considerations.

You are only one of seven billion human beings on this planet. To put that in perspective, imagine standing in the Rose Bowl completely packed with people in the seats and on the field. That would not even come close to being one in a million. Each of us is no more than a drop of rain in the torrent of life; nonetheless, there is no doubt of our value as individuals, because we are all important in some corner of destiny. The ultimate measure of our worth is how much we contribute to the welfare and success of those who accompany us on this brief journey through time while occupying this incredibly tiny ball in space. Go out and look up at the stars some night and remember that it takes over four years for light to travel to or from the star nearest our sun. We are tiny creatures in a huge universe, and we must take care of each other. It is terribly important that we look outside of ourselves to the needs of our neighbors.

The principles that have guided my life are not onerous and do not impose shackles that make living intolerable. They can, in fact, be summarized as succinctly as they were centuries ago and as I have repeatedly pointed out in this book, "Do unto others as you would have others do unto you"—something I first learned in Sunday school. I have read about morality, observed people's moral and immoral behaviors, thought about moral issues, and prayed about moral questions for my whole life. On reflection, I cannot honestly say that in doing so, I have learned anything profoundly superior or more important about the subject than I learned at the knees of Mr. Sebastian and my other Sunday school teachers all those years ago. I wish I could tell you that I have unfailingly followed that golden rule throughout my life. But I, like the other members of our species, have not. I have consciously and diligently tried to live by that simple command and will do so until the end. I have also tried hard to avoid the utter hypocrisy of espousing proper moral values while ignoring them in practice. I hope you will try your best to do so as well. The motto of the Alpha Omega Alpha Honorary Medical Society is "Be worthy to serve the suffering." Good luck in your career, and may God bless you for devoting yourself to serve those who suffer.

*I would thank you from the bottom of my heart,
but for you my heart has no bottom.*

—Author unknown

Chapter 14

Acknowledgments

Success in life is a group project; and any success that I have enjoyed I owe to those who have given me their love, support, and good works. That being so, this ought to be the longest chapter of the book because so many have helped me at one time or another. I will do my best to keep it short by applying group hugs where I can.

Where does one begin when giving thanks? I suppose I should start with my parents for taking the chance of having me in the first place and with all my teachers who opened the world and gave me a grand tour. From there, I have to dash to my beloved Arline, who has given me her undying devotion and help for the half century that we have known each other and been in love. I cannot forget my children, grandchildren, and sons-in-law, who have contributed in so many ways to make life happy, rewarding, and interesting. Being a devoted husband, father, and grandfather have been the greatest honors of my life. I love you all. No one goes through life alone, and I could not have done it without all these.

I am also grateful to all the physicians, nurse anesthetists, nurses, paramedics, and all other health care personnel with whom I have been honored and privileged to work during my training and practice. I include among these the members of the Ophthalmic Anesthesia Society, with whom I have been closely associated for more than twenty years. Karen Morgan and Bob Wagoner of AMA, Inc., who managed OAS during those years, were more helpful to the organization and me than I can possibly describe. My colleagues are too numerous to name, but if we have worked together, you know who you are. I have been blessed to know and work with an incredible group of skilled, compassionate, intelligent, caring, and selfless individuals during my career. The small number of "rotten apples" I mentioned in this book pale in comparison with all the rest. What a marvelous gift it has been to work with you all. My walking companions on the road of life have been extraordinary. I am especially grateful to Lynn Hauser and Neil Ross, who took a chance on hiring me at age fifty-one and gave me opportunities beyond my wildest dreams, including introducing me to Bob Hustead and Roy Hamilton, the two marvelous mentors who taught me ophthalmic anesthesia. I have been blessed in so many ways and by so many people that I can only say, "Thanks be to God!"

I owe special thanks to the best friend of my life other than my wife and children. The Reverend F. Paul Goodland was undoubtedly the most holy and yet most human individual I have been privileged to know. His unshakable faith, good humor, respect for others, and passionate work ethic are unforgettable to me. He stands out in my mind as a superb example of what it means to live a life devoted to Christ. He died over five years ago, but I still miss him.

The last thing I ever thought of doing in college was writing anything. In the fall of 2010, I became inflamed with the idea of sharing some of my most influential experiences in life with others. On a train trip to Chicago to attend the annual meeting of the Ophthalmic Anesthesia Society, ideas flashed in my mind and wrote themselves somewhere on my cerebral hemispheres, remaining entrenched on those feeble gyri until I could get home to my computer. Getting the essence written down initially was easy; and then the hard work of rewriting, editing, adding, and critiquing began. Putting little black letters onto white paper is not so challenging. Making those letters tell stories in a grammatically acceptable fashion turns out to be daunting, even for someone with a bit of writing and editing experience. I needed the help of others.

I owe so much to those who have assisted and supported me in the preparation of this book, including members of my family who made valuable and candid suggestions. Gabriele Roden, MD, a friend from the Ophthalmic Anesthesia Society and herself an author, helped me in several ways. Her book, *Behind the Ether Screen: Memoirs of an Anesthesiologist* (iUniverse, Bloomington, 2009), was an inspiration for me to start examining my past and begin organizing the experiences that have had the most profound effects on me. Her simple suggestions on improving my writing were superb and reminded me of my days in English composition classes as a freshman college student. After so many years, such help was sorely needed. Pat Reinhart, RN, is a nursing educator and friend at church. Her valuable comments and support have been greatly appreciated. Steffi Musa, RN, and Robin Hoyt, RN—both nurses at the Davis Duehr Dean Eye Surgery Center—were kind enough to read the manuscript and make excellent comments. Rachael Latchana, a college student, and Adam Quest, a fourth-year medical student at the time, graciously read the manuscript for me and made helpful remarks as well. Dr. Quest suggested the quotes by George Washington and Charles Austin Beard that appear in chapter 7, both of which seemed to fit perfectly the points I wished to raise. I am also indebted to Barry Jones, CRNA, another member of the Ophthalmic Anesthesia Society, who recommended the book by T. R. Reid cited in chapter 7. I knew Barry as an inhalation therapist in Iowa long before he went to nursing school and then became a CRNA. We met again years later at a society meeting. He now practices in South Dakota. Finally, I thank Fr. John Peters, whose friendship, support, and positive comments are so important to me.

Writing a book is a daunting task, but it pales in comparison with getting one's work published. I am so grateful to everyone at Xlibris for holding my hand during the process. I am especially indebted to my submissions representative, Cherry Minosa, for her guidance and support. The copyediting staff did a superb job of correcting the text without changing my intended meanings in any way. Thank you all for helping a true amateur share his thoughts and experiences with others.

Finally, I thank the nearly fifty thousand men, women, and children who honored me by trusting me with their lives and vision during the past forty-five years. I am humbled to think that so many people have placed their faith in me. It has truly been a privilege to serve each of them.

Made in the USA
San Bernardino,
CA